D1421471

The enterprise culture and
the inner city

Throughout the 1980s and into the 1990s, policy for inner city regeneration underwent a transformation from a reliance on central and local government activity and the use of public funds to a much heavier dependence on private sector activities and private investment. This new strategy was based on a conviction on the part of government that the 'engine of enterprise' could achieve in the inner cities what local government had so signally failed to do. It consisted of using public resources as incentives to attract commerce, business and industry back to designated sectors in or near to inner city areas. Regeneration would be development-led; enterprise activity would burgeon in the old wastelands; new jobs would be created; the 'inner city economies' would be revitalised and a dependent population energised by the culture of enterprise.

The Enterprise Culture and the Inner City evaluates the effectiveness of this strategy in alleviating urban deprivation. By examining four case studies – two Urban Development Corporations, one local government – private sector, and one purely private development – the authors make detailed analyses of job creation, 'leverage' (the ratio of public incentive to private investment funds), impact on local residents and the 'trickle effect' from enterprise down to the urban deprived.

The study is especially valuable as the fruit of independent scholarship, rather than funded research, in which the authors are able to offer a vigorously critical investigation of government policy. By taking into account the result of the 1992 general election and the implications of the Olympia & York Canary Wharf project, Nicholas Deakin and John Edwards present a credible prediction for the future (or lack of future) of the inner city.

The Enterprise Culture and the Inner City will be essential reading for students and lecturers of social and public policy and social science, professionals and lecturers in planning, and central and local government administrators.

Nicholas Deakin is Professor of Social Policy and Administration at the University of Birmingham, and **John Edwards** is Reader in Social Policy at the University of London.

The enterprise culture and the inner city

Nicholas Deakin and John Edwards

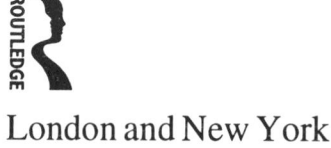

London and New York

First published in 1993
by Routledge
11 New Fetter Lane, London EC4P 4EE

Simultaneously published in the USA and Canada
by Routledge
29 West 35th Street, New York, NY 10001

© 1993 Nicholas Deakin and John Edwards

Typeset in Times by LaserScript Limited, Mitcham, Surrey
Printed and bound in Great Britain by
Mackays of Chatham PLC, Chatham, Kent.

British Library Cataloguing in Publication Data

A catalogue record for this book is available from the British Library.

Library of Congress Cataloging in Publication Data

Deakin, Nicholas.
The enterprise culture and the inner city/by Nicholas Deakin and John Edwards.
    p.   cm.
    Includes bibliographical references and index.
    1. Urban policy – Great Britain.   2. Inner cities – Great Britain.
    I. Edwards, John, 1943 Oct. 27–
    HT133.D43   1993
    307.3′42016′0941–dc20   92-28813
                                                                          CIP

ISBN: 0–415–03548–1
        0–415–03549–X (pbk)

To Lucy and Bridget

Contents

Illustrations

MAPS

TABLES

Preface

This is a book about 'those Inner Cities' (as Margaret Thatcher called them on the morning after the General Election of 1987). It is far from being the first and is unlikely to be the last. Previous books have addressed the complex tangle of issues comprehended under the label 'inner cities' in a variety of different ways and at an almost infinite number of levels. The range extends from the products of a massive research programme funded by the Economic and Social Research Council, which produced a shelf full of solid academic studies, to angry pamphlets published by community groups, sick of being the subjects of scrutiny and wishing to set their own agendas for discussion and action.

Why have we added to this lengthy – at times, it seems, never ending – procession of publications? There are two reasons. The first is to do with the nature of inner city policies. During the 1980s claims began to be heard that the 'problem' was at last on the way to being solved. The basis for this claim lay in the activities of the Urban Development Corporations, functioning as the instruments of what had come to be called the 'enterprise culture'. But although their activities had generated a great deal of publicity, had been celebrated in a number of glossy booklets issued by the government and were the subject of a cascade of consultants' reports, conclusive evidence – in the form of hard proof that claims were soundly based – proved curiously hard to locate. Our objective in undertaking the study was to get beneath the surface froth and to try to establish the basis on which the 'enterprise solution' was being advanced and how much substance there was in the claims being made for it.

In order to do so, we chose initially to undertake two case-studies in areas in which contrasting approaches had been adopted – one a straightforward example of the 'single minded' development agency and the other a collaboration between the local authority and the private sector. These were the Urban Development Corporation in Trafford Park near Manchester, and the Urban Development Authority in East Birmingham, known as Heartlands. We supplemented the material we collected in these two sites by observation and interview and eventually extended the analysis in two other directions; first, by assembling and analysing some of the copious material about the earliest and best known Development Corporation in the London Docklands; and second, by exploring what we have chosen to call a 'pure private' initiative, the Trafford Centre. These case-studies form the core of our book.

The second reason for undertaking this study is that both authors have in the past had direct personal experience of the operation of inner city policies – Nicholas Deakin as a local government officer and John Edwards as expert witness at a major planning inquiry. They have also previously collaborated on another study, together with Joan Higgins and Malcolm Wicks, in which they explored developments during earlier stages of inner city policy (Higgins *et al.* 1983). The authors now set out to build on that study and their own past involvement in an attempt to analyse the processes that have been at work in this latest (and highly distinctive) phase of inner city policy.

Finally, it is important to stress that this is not an official study; we have neither applied for nor been offered funding of any kind from any agency or institution, governmental or otherwise. Our sole means of extra support has been a grant of £552 that Nicholas Deakin received from a fund maintained by the Faculty of Commerce and Social Science in the University of Birmingham to pay for incidental expenses, which he gratefully acknowledges. Apart from this we could legitimately claim that this book is an independent product of our own unaided labours. But to do so would be to overlook the very helpful (and unconditional) assistance that we have received at all stages from those working in the field, at every level. Individual acknowledgements are made separately; but we could not have undertaken the study without such cooperation, for which we are most grateful. Nevertheless, our analysis remains the work of two outsiders, with all that this implies, both positively and in terms of lack of direct involvement in the policy-making process.

The text of this study remains substantially as it was submitted to the publishers in the Autumn of 1991; but the implications of a number of subsequent events are too important not to be touched on, however briefly and superficially. The opportunity has therefore been taken to update two of the case studies: London Docklands, by covering some of the immediate consequences of the collapse of the London property market, and in particular the impact on Olympia & York's flagship scheme at Canary Wharf; and in Birmingham Heartlands the constitutional changes leading to the declaration of an Urban Development Corporation (UDC). The result of the 1992 General Election, unexpected as it was to many people at the time, did at least have the merit (from the authors' perspective) of extending the period of relative stability in policy making – and hence, indirectly, the relevance of the conclusions reached in this study.

Finally, for the record, the division of labour on the writing of the study was as follows: John Edwards is responsible for Chapters 1, 2, 4, 5, 8 and 9. Nicholas Deakin wrote Chapters 6, 7 and 10. Chapters 3 and 11 are collaborations.

John Edwards, Egham – St Jean D'Aulps
Nicholas Deakin, Birmingham

Acknowledgements

In a book written without official sponsorship, the assistance of those involved in the design and implementation of inner city policies could not be taken for granted. This is why we are particularly grateful for the help freely given by a wide range of people, particularly in our case-study areas. Among them, Nicholas Deakin would especially like to name Sir Reginald Eyre, Alan Osborne, Jim Beeston and Monica Foot (Birmingham Heartlands). Elizabeth Filkin was also helpful at the initial stages of gathering information about London Docklands, as was Bob Colenutt at a later point.

John Edwards in turn wishes to acknowledge the assistance (and patience) of Mike Shields, Nick Gerrard, Ken Turner and others at the Trafford Park Development Corporation, and of Ian Betts who gave invaluable guidance through two planning inquiries and helped to make sense of the Dumplington Story. Thanks are also due to colleagues at Royal Holloway and Bedford New College for their support. None of these people are in any way responsible for errors of fact or eccentricities of interpretation.

Nicholas Deakin would also like to thank colleagues at the University of Birmingham for their tolerance during the period over which the research was being conducted: the Faculty of Commerce and Social Science's small research grant scheme enabled him to meet some of the incidental costs of the study. St Antony's College, Oxford, kindly offered Nicholas Deakin facilities for writing up his research as a Senior Associate Member – unfortunately illness prevented him from taking full advantage of the opportunity.

For both authors, family acknowledgements have been made elsewhere in different currency.

1 Enterprise as policy

In the period since 1980 the rationale underlying government policies for the inner cities has undergone a sea change.

Policies themselves have been radically transformed, partly in response to this change but also in deference to the explicit ideological predilections of the government. Such has been the presentation and packaging of these policies that it has not always been possible to distinguish the substantive from the illusory, but that there has been a real redirection of policy (and resources) is beyond doubt.

What has happened is that the enterprise culture has come to the inner cities. The idea that 'inner city problems' (whatever they may be) can be solved or even alleviated by targeting public resources into them in order to establish projects that will meet 'special' or 'additional' needs is now defunct. Once the 1977 White Paper *Policy for the Inner Cities* had put down a marker that the fundamental problem was the collapse of the economic infrastructures of the inner cities, the way was clear for an incoming government, ideologically so inclined, to see economic regeneration as a job for the private sector. Thus there was a neat fit between economic logic and ideological leanings. Clearly, only the private sector could produce the jobs and economic buoyancy that the inner cities lacked, and equally self-evident was the superior drive, energy and effectiveness of a private sector increasingly fired by the enterprise culture.

The engine of enterprise is now the driving force of inner city policies, and has been for some seven years. It is the purpose of this book to evaluate the enterprise strategy. At its simplest, our task is to answer the question, 'does the enterprise solution work?', but before we can begin to answer that we shall have to clarify a number of other questions. How much of the overall solution to inner city problems is it claimed the enterprise strategy will provide? What are inner city problems (not so arcane a question as it looks) and which ones might the enterprise strategy have an impact on and which must find other solutions? What is the logic of the enterprise solution; how does it solve inner city problems? There will be many other questions to answer along the way and many different versions of success to tease out, but in essence our purpose is a simple one: a radically different strategy to deal with the inner cities has been in full gear for more than half a decade; does it work?

The ideas of enterprise and the enterprise culture are of course chimeric; they are as much prescriptive rallying slogans as descriptions of cogent concepts, but the policy changes they have wrought are real enough and we cannot ignore that these are inextricably tied to the sets of attitudes and beliefs that characterise those who promote enterprise. Inner city policies have changed *because* of the sets of attitudes that go to make up the enterprise culture and these attitudes in turn have informed policy. We cannot therefore understand the directional drive of current inner city policies without an understanding of what 'enterprise' and the 'enterprise culture' mean.

'Enterprise' in the political lexicon of the 1980s is a property exclusive to the private sector. The public sector does not possess it, or worse, it is a hindrance to its exercise. But it is also shorthand for a collection of other, related values, values which, as Corner and Harvey note, are ' . . . primarily, to do with the economics of neo-liberal "freedom" and the politics of individualism' (Corner and Harvey 1990: 24). Enterprise is having initiative and drive; it is taking opportunities when they arise; it is independence from the state; it is having confidence and being responsible for one's own destiny; it is being driven by the work ethic; and it promotes self-interest. But it is in this last property that its real value as a policy instrument lies. There is no stronger motivating force, so the culture of enterprise tells us, than the pursuit of self-interest. This is what gets things done. Why not therefore harness this, the strongest motive to action, to serve your policy goals? True it is unlikely that effective action will be directed precisely at your policy goals, but if these can be effected as an intended (on the government's part) or unintended (on the part of the entrepreneur) consequence of being enterprising, then you will have achieved your policy goals and at minimum cost to the public purse. Furthermore, the drive of enterprise will have achieved at little cost what countless millions of public expenditure has failed to achieve.

It is just this sort of reasoning (only mildly parodied here) that lies behind the drive to bring enterprise to the inner cities.

More than this however, the enterprise culture was (and remains) an integral part of the government's philosophy. It was, as Corner and Harvey point out, not simply descriptive but also, and mainly, a campaigning idea (Corner and Harvey 1990: 24), a set of beliefs that permeated the government's approach to everything it was doing (with the possible exception of foreign policy). In other words, the enterprise culture was at the heart of the cultural revolution that the government saw as necessary before economic recovery and national pride would be re-established. To this extent, there was nothing unique about the inner cities (though they were singled out by the then Prime Minister on election night in 1987). Quite simply, they, like most things, would benefit from the latent energy that commitment to the enterprise culture would release.

There was, however, one train of events that made inner city problems seem peculiarly vulnerable to the enterprise approach. Until 1977 or thereabouts, if there was any consensus (or indeed any cogent view at all) about the nature and causes of urban deprivation (as the inner cities problem was then more usually styled), it was that inner city areas contained disproportionately large concentrations of the poor, the dependent and the inadequate. To this could be added a poor physical environment, poor housing and a lack of social and community facilities. Urban deprivation was essentially a residual problem of the welfare state (Lawless 1979; Edwards 1984). The policy response (mainly by means of the Urban Programme, the Educational Priority Areas, Section 11 Grant and the Community Development Projects)[1] was to target more (or re-directed) resources into these areas to provide for the additional and special needs to be found there. For reasons that we shall discuss at greater length in Chapter 2, this diagnosis was transformed over a relatively short period (very approximately between 1975 and 1978) and there emerged the new orthodoxy that the root cause of the problems of the inner cities was the collapse of their economic infrastructures brought about by the emigration of firms to out-of-town sites or their death *in situ*, compounded by the socially selective emigration of their populations (see Hall *et al.* 1973; Elias and Keogh 1982; Lawless and Brown 1986; Manners 1986; Robson 1988). What needed to be done was now clear: new industry, new jobs, and an economically active population had to be attracted back into the inner areas in order to regenerate their economic infrastructures. It was a diagnosis that lent itself far more readily than its predecessor to an enterprise culture solution. And the timing was just about right. The new diagnosis received official confirmation in the 1977 White Paper and a government committed to the enterprise response came to power two years later.

REALITY AND ILLUSION

Even a cursory glance at government inner city brochures since 1987 is all that is required to see that there has been a strong presentational element in the way in which policy information is conveyed. These are no longer policy statements so much as hortatory notices of progress and intent. Their style allows of no debate or dissension any more than the sales brochures of property developers. The style and language is that of the enterprise culture and the purpose has been less to inform than to promote the 'enterprise revolution'. The problem with presentational politics, however, is that it engenders cynicism and distrust. If the way government presents its policies has the superficial gloss of a Sunday colour supplement there must always be the suspicion that the content is equally insubstantial. We are left wondering how much of current policy and recent policy change has real substance and how much is old policy decked out in presentational froth. (The answer, it turns out, is 'a good deal of substance' as we shall see, but we ought certainly to be forgiven for harbouring some doubts.)

The launch of *Action for Cities* was an example *par excellence* of the triumph of packaging over substance. The purpose was to launch a new 'drive' on the inner cities and the occasion was a press conference attended by the Prime Minister with six ministers-in-attendance, each armed with a copy of the *Action for Cities* brochure (Cabinet Office 1988). The message was exclusively that regenerating the inner cities was a job for the private sector and that local authorities would be relegated to a minor role in which the damage they could do could be controlled. The sub-text however was, in all significant respects, a panegyric to the enterprise culture and this appeared to be an important – if not the most important – part of the exercise. No new policies were announced, the then Prime Minister herself admitting 'It is not a new programme. I don't think there's a single new policy here' (as reported in the *Guardian* 8 March 1988) but rather, a bringing together of all existing policies under a new umbrella. But neither was any new co-ordinative machinery on offer, so that the 'bringing together' was collectivisation in name only though it did permit, by the inclusion of education, crime, tourism and a number of other activities, a new global sum of £3,000m for inner city policies to be floated.

However, it has to be said that if the purpose of this kind of presentational politics has been to inculcate the *idea* of enterprise as an effective policy agent then it has in many respects been successful. Whether or not it works (something it is our purpose to examine in this book), the *idea* of the usefulness and even the necessity of the private sector as an instrument of regeneration is now firmly planted, and policy has followed in the wake of this conviction. Therefore, whilst presentational politics combined with an *apparent* lack of substantial change in policy give an impression of the power of packaging over content, the reality is quite different and it may be that government policy presentation has done a disservice, less in cloaking old policies in glossy covers than in engendering an impression of the insubstantial when what is on offer is very substantial. We devote Chapter 3 to a detailed examination of how policy changed over a period of twelve years from an emphasis on service provision to one of economic regeneration, but in essence what has happened has been a reorientation of existing policies and a redirection of finance to promote the enterprise culture rather than the generation of entirely new policies. This may in part account for the impression of a victory of presentation over substance, but the shift of emphasis has been real and inner city policies of the early 1990s are very different from those of the previous decade.

However, the story is not a straightforward one. Policy development and the promotion of enterprise have not always moved forward in tandem. The idea of urban development corporations for example, which the government now presents as the spearhead of the enterprise attack on the inner cities, was first given reality (in the form of the London Docklands and Merseyside Development Corporations) in 1981, yet it was six years before it was brought to the forefront of inner city policy. Indeed, so many and so apparently fleeting have been the shifts in policy over the past decade that it is often difficult to identify any coherent strategy. There are at present, for example, thirty-two schemes directed solely or in large measure at the inner cities (see Chapter 3, p. 55–6) and all fall loosely under the *Action for Cities* umbrella. ('Loosely' because there is no definitive list).[2] It is not surprising therefore that *Action for Cities* should engender confusion or that some of these schemes occasionally 'disappear', only to surface again when the need arises. Nor, given this multiplicity of schemes should it be surprising if there appears to be little coherence to the overall strategy (if, indeed, there were an overall strategy). The story is not a simple one to tell therefore, and we should not expect to find an unhindered line of policy development leading to the enthronement of enterprise. When the House of Commons Public Accounts Committee produced its report on regenerating the inner cities in 1990, it accepted the view of the Department of the Environment that there could not be any 'master plan' but it still had difficulty making sense of 'this recipe for confusion and overlap' (House of Commons 1990: V).

There is another reason why inner city policy has at times been difficult to comprehend and that is that prime responsibility for it (more accurately, them) appears to have floated from one department to another. The Department of the Environment first took over responsibility from the Home Office in 1976 but with the shift in emphasis from social provision to economic regeneration and skills-development, the Departments of Trade and Industry and of Employment have played an increasingly prominent role over which Environment has not seen fit, or has not been able, to exercise hegemony. There has not therefore, in recent years, as the Public Accounts Committee note, been any single department with overall responsibility for all inner city policies (House of Commons 1990: VI).

There has, however (to add to the confusion), been an 'inner cities minister' responsible for the presentation of policies but this ministerial position has not rested with any one department. The position was first held by Mr Kenneth Clarke at Employment; he was followed by Mr Tony Newton at Trade and Industry and then, in the Summer of 1989, by Mr David Hunt at Environment.

What is now being done at the beginning of the 1990s by way of inner city policy therefore is very different from what was done a decade earlier. There *has* been a fundamental shift even though the names of some of the policy components are now a decade old, despite the heavy rhetorical overlay and despite the absence of a coherent longer-term strategy. Behind the sometimes illusory gloss of the enterprise culture, different ends are being pursued and money is being spent in different ways. And all this will affect – for good or ill – people who live in the inner cities. But their welfare on the one hand and successful economic regeneration on the other may not necessarily be synonymous.

EVALUATING THE ENTERPRISE APPROACH

There are two broad themes to our evaluation of the enterprise approach to the inner cities and each has a number of components. The first concerns the logic of economic regeneration as a means of reducing or eliminating urban deprivation – which we take to be the human component of the inner city problem. To put it at its starkest, how do the glittering (or tawdry) towers of docklands reduce poverty and privation? This will require us to assess the 'reach' of regeneration into the social conditions in the inner cities but also the wisdom of trying to reverse history – of trying to recreate what policy rhetoric appears to assert were the culturally rich, vital and throbbing cores of our cities – devoid (presumably) of poverty and hardship. The second theme revolves around some important consequences of adopting a private enterprise approach and, in particular, the change in the principal actors responsible for implementing policy including the relative exclusion of local government, and the effects these changes have on the accountability for policies and their outcomes. If, for example, responsibility for putting inner city policy into practice shifts either wholly or on balance from local government to private sector developers and financial markets, who then is to be accountable for policy outputs and to whom? Once more, to put it at its starkest, who is to be held accountable (and to whom) if economic regeneration fails and inner city residents are left no better, or worse off? Or, more problematically, who is to be held accountable (and to whom) if economic regeneration *succeeds* and inner city residents are left no better, or worse off?

Urban deprivation and economic regeneration

An imperative of any policy is that there must be some causal connection between what it is doing, and what it is meant to achieve. Such a connection is not immediately obvious in the case of current inner city policies for two reasons. First, recent policy 'statements' have been determinedly reticent on the issue of what is to be achieved. And second, if we take the liberty of assuming that part, at least, of what is to be achieved is a diminution of urban deprivation and if we permit ourselves to think that this includes reductions in poverty, privation and dependency, then it is not manifestly clear how economic regeneration will affect these issues.

Our evaluation therefore will require us to specify in detail what constitutes the 'inner city problem'. We shall find that there is a multiplicity of components including economic, social and physical ones, and it is the second of these that will prove to be the most testing for the economic regeneration strategy. Among the social indicators, the incidence of which will be found to be relatively greater in inner city areas, will be poverty, unemployment and dependency, particularly among the elderly, the young and the chronically sick. These constitute an important part of urban deprivation (itself a part of the inner city problem). Two lines of approach then present themselves for our evaluation of policy in respect of these characteristics. The first is whether and how the economic regeneration strategy itself may reach down to impact upon them. The second is to see what, if any, other components of the overall inner city policy package may have an impact on them and this will require also that we assess the extent to which the other (and lesser) parts of the strategy are compatible with, and additive to, the economic regeneration component. The more problematic of the two lines of approach however is undoubtedly the first. It is easy enough to see how service provision can alleviate privation; it is not so clear how private sector investment in an area will do so. Certainly, insofar as greater employment prospects are a necessary component of relieving deprivation, then inward investment which produces jobs that go to the presently unemployed will be beneficial, but how far such benefit will 'trickle down' to those not in the labour market remains to be investigated. Some private sector investment for job creation must therefore be a part of the policy package but it will be of benefit, even to those in the labour market, only if this market is manipulated in such a way as to ensure that they get the jobs.

Reversing history

The strategy is one of economic *re*generation. It is a strategy (presumably) to restore the inner cities to some former state which (again presumably) was one of economic vitality and social well-being. However, there are some weighty, and usually unspoken, assumptions behind the wisdom and efficacy of trying to recreate the right mix of economic activity and population profiles which (we are expected to believe) worked before the 'great decline'. Were the areas we call inner cities once of such a nature that we are right in wanting now to recreate them? Two aspects of this question immediately present themselves. Firstly, how much of a mix was there in the pre-decline inner cities of economic and social activity; how socially heterogeneous were they; and did manufacturing and commercial activities sit happily with residential usage? Secondly, the regeneration thesis does assume that the inner cities were social and economic microcosms with their own relatively self-contained economies. If this was ever the case, is there reason to believe that it could or would be the case now or in the future? Or is it as plausible for example to promote the inner cities as (say) purely residential areas (or for that matter, as purely industrial or commercial locations)? There are two uncertainties that should at least give us reason to entertain such possibilities. The first is whether economic activity (of whatever kind) has to be in the inner cities to be of benefit to them. The second is whether we have any more reason to believe that inner city residents wish to live in close proximity to non-residential land users than do their suburban counterparts. After all, does it make any more sense in an age of international corporatism to speak of inner city economies than it does to entertain the idea of suburban economies? Are there inner city economies that can be regenerated? We must, at the very least, countenance the possibility that reversing history might not work.

A question of areas

Reversing history carries another implicit assumption about the spatial discreteness of the inner cities. It has a number of components, the most significant of which for our purposes are that inner city areas *are* spatially discrete areas; that the deprived are concentrated in spatially discrete areas; that there is such a thing as an inner city economy and that, in consequence, the policy strategy of area designations is an appropriate one.

An evaluation of the rationale of economic regeneration and of its effectiveness will require us (in a way that other inner city policies do not) to subject these assumptions to more critical scrutiny.

There is an arbitrary answer to the question of the spatial insularity of the inner city (or of inner city areas) and one that area designation *ipso facto* uses, and that is simply to draw boundaries on a map. But it hardly needs saying that this will neither necessarily nor usually define functionally discrete areas or separate spatial economies or exclusive concentrations of deprived people. Indeed, it is the very arbitrariness of area designations that is in question. We shall not delay long over the question of how detached inner cities are, because this resolves itself into the more refined question of how spatially discrete are the concentrations of the various components that go to make up the inner city problem *in combination*. In other terms this means that we are concerned with whether and to what extent components such as social deprivation, physical decay, poor housing and absence of local jobs occur together in concentration. (There is another aspect to this of course which we shall not be able to answer and that is, how *much* of *all* deprivation, physical decay, bad housing and economic stagnation will be captured and dealt with by strategies of area designation in urban areas?)

The danger in adopting such an 'essential' approach is that you simply raise more questions than you can answer – and not a few that are unanswerable given the paucity of adequate data. None the less, there is need for an antidote to the before-and-after photographs that have passed for evaluation in recent years. A good deal – and probably most – of present inner city strategy including the Urban Programme, Urban Development Corporations, Task Forces, City Action Teams, Enterprise Zones and a number of others, relies on area designation and assumes the existence of relatively insulated areas of social, physical and economic decay. Such a strategy presents few problems if needs are identified in an area and resources targeted there to meet them. But this says nothing about whether this is an appropriate way of meeting most needs. Even less self-evident is the logic of meeting needs (urban deprivation) by attracting whatever investment you can into a defined area in the expectation of reviving an 'inner city economy' (that perhaps never existed), the benefits of which will trickle downwards and outwards to the aid of the needy. It may work, but the social and economic logic involved is not immediately compelling.

Partnerships and alliances

Traditionally, inner city policies have involved central government as grant giver and local authorities as recipient and spender (along with varying degrees of voluntary sector involvement) and this arrangement has continued to the present for those authorities which do not have partnership status. For the partnership authorities however (first designated in 1977), the relationship between central and local government became, in theory at least, more formalised. For them, there was to be a partnership operation with central government to be effected through partnership committees consisting of representatives of central and local government, local health authorities and the Manpower Services Commission and to be chaired by a minister. The purpose of the arrangement was to develop *jointly* a three-year programme of expenditure that would have a coherence that the original Urban Programmes lacked (being essentially a money-dispensing machine). The emphasis was to be on the co-ordination of the activities of participating bodies through the mechanism of the Partnership Committees (see Higgins *et al.* 1983: 175 *et seq.*). And co-ordination, as we shall see, has remained a concern of inner city policy implementation ever since. The idea of partnership has also survived to the present day but the partners have changed.

Once the private sector has been cast in the role of policy instrument new alliances have to be made, not only because there is a new actor on the stage but primarily because, to be effective, private sector effort must be harnessed or exploited. For the purposes of our evaluation of enterprise in the inner cities we shall examine, by way of case-studies, two types of partnership arrangement involving the private sector, one involving central government, the other, local government.

The Urban Development Corporations, though necessarily having to deal with local authorities ('cooperate' would not, in some and perhaps most cases, be an accurate description of the relationship), are in effect an arrangement between the private sector and central government. To all intents and purposes the arrangement is one whereby the development corporation uses central government (and its own) funds in order to attract investment to its designated area by means of subsidies, tax holidays and the provision of infrastructure. (Their position as the spearhead of government strategy for the inner cities is testified to by the 61 per cent share of total inner city expenditure they took in 1990–1 (Department of the Environment 1990a).)

The salient feature of Urban Development Corporations (which were modelled on the New Town Development Corporations (Schaffer 1972; Aldridge 1979; Heseltine 1987)) is perhaps that they are not local authorities. In 1981 the government saw fit to fashion these new 'single-minded' agencies to do a job of which it thought local authorities incapable. Their function has been to act as an interface between central government and the private sector, both facilitating private investment and welding this to the service of central government strategy for inner city regeneration. It is through the development corporations that the partnership (or perhaps alliance) between central government and the private sector is put into action. The strategy is not without its hazards however – and not least because being market-led it is subject to the vicissitudes of boom and recession, particularly in the property market. Our concern must be therefore not only whether private sector investment (whether manufacturing, commercial or property) can reach down to urban deprivation as we have outlined above, but also whether a strategy that is subject to market fluctuations can provide the longer-term stability and continuity that is required for the job of economic *and social* regeneration to be done.

An alliance between local government and the private sector as an instrument of policy is not a part of the government's strategy for the inner cities. Indeed, given the government's pronounced lack of confidence in local government in general and Labour-controlled authorities in particular, and its intermittent attempts to cut them out of inner city policies, such an alliance must seem to be the least likely to produce any effect at all. Was it not just because of the alleged antipathy of Labour local authorities (and not a few Conservative ones too) to anything with the slightest taint of enterprise, that urban development corporations had to be created? Yet the experience of Heartlands in Birmingham which we examine in Chapter 7 demonstrates that what is 'unthinkable' is only unthinkable to those with certain ideological tunnel vision. Heartlands, like several of our other case-studies, is in its infancy (indeed, apart from the London and Merseyside docklands, all the private sector alliances in the inner cities are recent creations) but it is far enough developed for us to see that its purpose and strategy are not greatly dissimilar to those of most urban development corporations. It is of particular interest to us however, because it sought to achieve broadly similar aims by means of a direct partnership between a number of large private sector institutions and Birmingham City Council. An evaluation of Heartlands and the progress made as a partnership will provide a valuable comparison with the achievements of development corporations, and one of our purposes here will be to assess whether what the private sector can provide is better harnessed by specially created 'single-minded' instruments or by direct partnership with a local authority.

There is a third alternative to alliance with central or local governments for the private sector. Again, it is not a part of government policy – indeed it is not a policy at all in any specific sense. It is just that the undirected, unsubsidised activities of private sector developers will, in certain circumstances, have an impact for good or ill on the inner cities.

We shall distinguish this activity from those circumstances in which the private sector forms a partnership or alliance with central or local government by calling it 'pure private' activity (though in practice it may turn out not to be very pure).

A necessary component of any strategy that attempts either to involve the private sector in regeneration by means of subsidies or ready-made infrastructure, or one that seeks to achieve the same end by the provision of grants for projects, is that it must involve the designation of a defined area as being one in which the subsidies or grants apply. Urban development corporations are charged with regenerating their designated area, inner area programmes apply in defined areas and Heartlands is a defined area. There will be many circumstances however in which developers of one sort or another will own land within designated areas or sufficiently proximate to them to be in their labour-draw area, or indeed in or close to any area of urban deprivation whether designated or not. Development of such land for commercial, retailing, leisure or manufacturing purposes will have some impact on the inner city areas and in many cases such impact will not differ in kind from that achieved by investment drawn to the area by subsidy or the attraction of a ready infrastructure.

There will be cases if such development land falls within a designated area that the owner will be able to make use of subsidies to carry out development, but there will be others (usually when development occurs outside the designated area) when the financial advantage of owning the land will far outweigh the benefit of subsidies, and development may go ahead in its 'pure private' form. Where such development does occur of course, it will not form part of any inner city strategy such as would exist in an urban development corporation; nor would it have attached to it any efforts to ensure that local people gained the benefit of new employment. But neither, as we demonstrate in subsequent chapters, does this always occur when efforts are made to promote it. Nor did the proscription in the 1988 Local Government Act of local labour clauses in local authority contracts with companies undertaking developments in inner city areas with public subsidy do anything to facilitate the allocation of jobs to local people. Indeed, it is largely because Section 17 of the act cuts so clearly across the grain of inner city policy that it is now being reviewed (see House of Commons 1990: 14). There is no reason however why the relevant local authority or authorities could not use such planning powers as they have to exploit such development for the benefit of their inner city areas. There is no reason, for example, why planning consents cannot be attached to requirements of good faith efforts to employ local people or to establish jointly-sponsored training programmes for the under-skilled. We shall examine a case of potential large scale development where imaginative exploitation by local authorities could have ensured such benefits for the inner city.

It is not possible to say with any degree of certainty how much potential 'pure private' development exists either within or close to inner city areas, but it is likely to be very considerable and may in total far exceed what can be drawn into designated areas by various forms of sweeteners. What is certainly the case is that it is a resource of great *potential* benefit to the inner cities that ought not to be ignored.

Accountability and participation

Much has been made of the fact that urban development corporations are unelected bodies (see Docklands Consultative Committee 1988; Lawless 1988a: 282; Nicholson 1989: 53; Batley 1989).

How much difference this really makes (and to whom) when compared with local authorities, however, is a matter of conjecture. Some development corporations have been sufficiently stung by criticisms of their lack of *local* accountability to have created consultative committees as a means by which the 'local community' can have its say in developments taking place. The local government–private sector alliance will not, on the other hand (in theory at least), be subject to such criticism because the local democratic machinery will still ensure accountability to the electorate. The same cannot be said of the 'pure private' solution except insofar as local authorities become involved in exploiting development and private developers are responsible (where relevant) to their shareholders. But then that has nothing to do with local accountability.

There are in fact two related issues involved here – accountability and participation. Urban development corporations are accountable – but only to Parliament. They have, however (some at least), made attempts to consult the local community and to enable it to participate in some decision making (though not, it has to be said, the important decisions). Contrariwise, a local authority is in theory locally accountable but it need neither consult nor participate with the local community. (In Heartlands, accountability remains in place but has been supplemented with varying degrees of consultation and participation (see Chapter 7).)

In any of the arrangements we consider in subsequent chapters, a necessary consequence of success must be that the lives of many people will be affected, and not all beneficially. We must consider therefore the extent and effectiveness of such accountability as there is to the affected population in the various arrangements, and the degree to which they are enabled to participate in deciding what should happen to them.

There is, however, a further aspect of accountability and participation that arises when the enterprise culture enters the policy equation, and it is one that so far has received little attention. The enterprise culture, we are told, turns us all from being clients, travellers, patients and users into customers. And customers, we are told, are more powerful than mere consumers or supplicants. If the enterprise culture comes to the inner cities therefore, might it be possible that it will bring with it the power of consumerism, not just in respect of people's relations to the providers of housing, leisure, public services and so on, but also in the more visceral sense of bringing the cultural revolution of enterprise? In short, can inner city residents become 'empowered' by consumerism in a way that community participation has failed to deliver for so long?

Public ends and private means

Using the private sector of the economy to pursue broadly social (or at least 'public') ends is not unique to inner city policy; nor is this the first time it has been so used (we have had regional development policies and industrial location policies since 1934 – see Cullingworth 1985), but present inner city policies are the first instance of an 'enterprise solution' to social problems. Whereas regional development or industrial location policies were concerned only with the geographical distribution of investment, something much more is expected of the private sector in the inner cities. There is, as we have noted, an unspecified but assumed rationale to present policy that private sector investment in the inner cities will do more than simply relocate economic activity; it will have far more penetrative effects into the social and economic life of inner urban areas. At least, this is how government brochures and development corporation publicity appear to see things. Whether private sector investors in the inner cities are themselves aware of the percolative role they are playing, however, is something we examine in subsequent chapters.

There is a broader question that present strategy raises however, and one that has relevance for social policy more generally. It is a question of the compatibility of public ends and private means. The purposes that private sector investors pursue are necessarily different from the ends we hope to achieve through social policies. They are not wholly incompatible however (if they were, the strategy as a whole would be a nonsense). The same results may be achieved by different purposes, but – superficially at least – it does look at though such *tangible* social benefits as may result are a by-product of actions taken for quite different reasons. (We leave aside here the less tangible 'benefit' of promoting the enterprise culture revolution.) Whilst it must be the case that private sector investment in inner city areas can potentially be of benefit to the deprived and dependent – an empirical issue – there remains a moral dimension to the use of private means for public ends. It is just this: should the welfare (in its broadest sense) of the poor and dependent be tied to a possibly fleeting coincidence of interests between public and private sectors? The present recession gives ample warning that the strategy may be all too dependent on fluctuations in property markets.

NOTES

1   There is a considerable literature on these various schemes. Evidence of the conception of urban deprivation that underpinned each of them may be found in Edwards and Batley 1978 (the Urban Programme); Halsey 1972 (the Educational Priority Areas); Greve 1973 (the Community Development Projects).

2   The National Audit Office report on inner cities in 1989 identified some thirty-four projects. Estimated numbers differ, partly because there is constant flux in programmes and partly as a result of ambiguity about whether particular programmes are directed primarily at the inner cities.

2 From public provision to private enterprise

THE PROBLEM RE-DIAGNOSED

The private enterprise 'solution' to the problem of the inner cities grew by fits and starts over a period of approximately a decade with the seeds being unwittingly sown in the mid-1970s. During this period (neither the beginning nor end of which can clearly be pinned down), the nature of inner city policy moved from public provision for 'additional' or 'special' needs to regeneration by private enterprise (albeit with a little help from public funds). In order to understand just how radical this shift of policy logic has been and how fundamentally the enterprise solution differs from preceding 'solutions', we use this chapter to chart the faltering steps on the way to the emergence of the private sector strategy as *the* predominant measure by which to 'turn around' the inner cities.

So far as possible, events are treated chronologically, but the non-linear nature of the shift from public provision to private enterprise makes a strictly chronological account both more difficult and less revealing.

During the 1980s two quite separate ideas converged that enabled the marriage of enterprise and the inner cities to take place. The first was a necessary, though unintended precursor to the idea of private sector led economic regeneration. It represented a reconstruction of the way in which the nature of the 'inner city problem' was perceived (Edwards 1984). Whilst it would impose too great a sense of coherence on thinking about inner cities in the 1960s and 1970s to suggest that there was any orthodoxy of view about the nature and causes of urban deprivation (a term much more in evidence then than now), it would be true to say that there was a greater convergence of ideas around the notion of concentrations of deprived people (for whatever reason) than on any other possible interpretation. (See for example some of the earlier analyses of the inner city problem such as those to be found in Lawless (1979) and Edwards and Batley (1978).) Inner city policies during these two decades were certainly predicated upon the idea of concentrations of deprived people. The Urban Programme (the main policy instrument during this period) and the later Community Development Projects were primarily concerned with 'additional' service provision and consciousness- and confidence-raising in deprived areas respectively (see Hatch *et al.* 1977; Community Development Project 1977a and b; Edwards and Batley 1978; Higgins *et al.* 1983). Early Urban Programme circulars for example characterised the 'inner city problem' and the nature of potential recipient areas in the following terms:

> 'Areas of special social need' means local areas. . . where living conditions are particularly poor. . . and pressure on social services is severe. Evidence of social need may take many forms – poverty; high levels of unemployment, delinquency, mental disorder or children in care; overcrowding, old and dilapidated housing; inadequate community services; a poor quality of environment. Many such areas have large concentrations of Commonwealth immigrants.
>
> (Home Office 1974:1)

There is nothing here about economic infrastructure and the need for economic regeneration as the *sine qua non* of the rebirth of the inner cities. Here was a traditional 'welfarist' response to what were perceived as concentrations of need. It was selectivity without (much) stigma; rather than select out needy people on the basis of a needs (means) test, the same – or at least a similar – end could be achieved by targeting the areas in which they seemed to be concentrated. Titmuss (and Edwards and Batley) called it, incorrectly, positive discrimination (Titmuss 1968: 135). It was nothing of the kind; it was resource allocation according to need but crudely targeted and in the end ineffectual.

Little was written or said during the 1960s and a large part of the 1970s to suggest that much thought had been given to the aetiology of deprivation, and it certainly did not inform policy debate. That there were concentrations of the poor and dependent was evident (that a greater number of the poor and dependent lived outside the inner city concentrations was less so), but why this should have been the case seemed to be something that did not tax the collective mind.[1]

The beginnings of the change that eventually enabled a 'free enterprise solution' to be brought to bear on the inner cities can be traced – ironically, given the predominant ideological complexion of those involved – to the accumulated reports of the twelve Community Development Projects established by that highly conservative government department, the Home Office, in 1969. This ground has been well tilled and we need not linger over it here (see for example Specht 1976; Higgins 1978; Loney 1981; Higgins *et al.* 1983: Chapter 2), but the cumulative message of the projects (much to the dismay of Home Office civil servants who saw their own role change from facilitators to experts in damage limitation) was that if there had been an unwritten leitmotiv to the work so far that characterised inner city residents as inadequate, unfortunate or – worst of all – that pulpit platitude 'those less fortunate', then not only was it inappropriate but it led to a policy blind-alley. There was a good deal of petticoat-flouncing among and between the Community Development Project (CDP) teams in those years (with Home Office civil servants rushing off to the nether parts of the kingdom to smooth them down), but what they provided, for the first time, was documented evidence of the nature and causes of the decline in their areas. And the story was the same from Hillfields in Coventry to Clarksfield in Oldham and from Benwell in Newcastle to Batley in the West Riding. There was a *reason* for the coincidence of physical decay and social deprivation; it was that the economic activity upon which the residents of these areas had depended so long for their livelihood had disappeared; either it had migrated elsewhere or it had died *in situ* (see in particular *Gilding the Ghetto* (Community Development Project 1977a) and *The Costs of Industrial Change* (Community Development Project 1977b)).

Whilst this was not a startling revelation (particularly to inner city residents) it was, for the first time in the CDP reports, documented with evidence and – most importantly – linked to a critique of then government policy, including the CDPs themselves. By the time *Gilding the Ghetto* and *The Costs of Industrial Change* appeared in 1977, the whole CDP enterprise was nearing the end of its life and the teams in the field were almost completely estranged from Home Office officials. Whereas some of the earlier CDP reports had been published with a Home Office *imprimatur* (and hence were graced with a semblance of officialdom), the Home Office disowned much of the later, more 'radical' output. Any direct impact that the CDP reports may have had on the policy process therefore is likely to have been a negative one. The Home Office was not about to take on board what some of its civil servants thought of as 'radical *chic*'. Yet by means that are probably untraceable, the CDP analysis did have an impact in the longer term. It may only have been at the level of informing the debate (it certainly did coincide with a noticeable shift in the focus of the academic literature). But the essential message – that making small additional welfare provisions for the residue of the unfortunate that the welfare state had not yet reached was misconceived, palliative and probably futile – was not lost. Inner city policy was anyway in upheaval at this time both in terms of thinking and strategy and of organisational responsibility. The CDP message was fed into the melting pot.

The transfer of responsibility for inner city policies from the Home Office to the Department of the Environment (a responsibility that the

Home Office was more than happy to relinquish) was the first of a number of moves, but it was one that was crucial to a shift in policy direction. The Home Office had never been a suitable home for the Urban Programme (UP) and the Community Development Projects; it had responsibility only because the origins of the UP lay in concerns about immigration and race relations, and by the mid-1970s it was acting as little more than a postbox for processing grant applications between other central departments and local authorities. Meanwhile, strategic thinking about the inner cities had passed to the Department of the Environment, where in 1972 Peter Walker had commissioned the three inner area studies in Lambeth, Liverpool and Birmingham, the general conclusions of which closely matched those of the CDP reports once the latter had been stripped of some of their more strident rhetoric (the most accessible output from the inner area studies are the three final reports (Department of the Environment 1977a, b and c) and the summary report (Department of the Environment 1977d)). The message, which found its way into the seminal White Paper of 1977, was that whatever the *manifestation* of deprivation, such as concentrations of the poor, deprived and dependent, the *reason* for these concentrations was socially selective population loss from the inner cities, leaving high proportions of the dependent and very high dependency ratios and the decline (and sometimes collapse) of the economic infrastructure of the areas. Thus began the long process by which enterprise came to the inner cities.

1977: THE STAMP OF APPROVAL

The new diagnosis (and really the first coherent diagnosis) of the reasons for the problems of the inner cities entered the policy arena via the 1977 White Paper *Policy for the Inner Cities* (Department of the Environment 1977e), by which time Labour was in power and Peter Shore was in charge at Environment. But if the new diagnosis lent itself to a policy strategy that sat more easily with Conservative rather than Labour ideology, no one seemed to notice at the time.

The White Paper drew directly on the three inner area studies for its characterisation of the problem to be tackled and the reasons for it. It then went on, under the heading *What Needs to be Done*:

> The first essential is a specific commitment on the part of central and local government to the regeneration of the inner areas. . . the underlying aims must include:
>
> a) strengthening the economies of the inner areas and the prospects of their residents;

   b) improving the physical fabric of the inner areas and making their environment more attractive;

   c) alleviating social problems;

   d) securing a new balance between the inner areas and the rest of the city region in terms of population and jobs.

(Department of the Environment 1977e: 25,26)

If the Urban Programme had had any coherent set of aims, the nearest equivalent on this list would be item c), the alleviation of social problems. Clearly, inner city policies were, after 1977, intended to be about much more.

The White Paper then went on to develop what needed to be done by way of 'economic improvement' to strengthen the economies of the inner areas:

> it is vital to preserve the firms and businesses which at present exist in the inner areas.
>
> indigenous growth needs to be cultivated by facilitating the expansion of local firms.
>
> New sites and premises. . . are needed in order to attract suitable manufacturing, service and office firms to settle within the cities.

(Department of the Environment 1977e: 27)

So here was the first policy step along the road to regeneration by enterprise. The language may be different, but the sentiments would be equally at home in today's inner city policies.

If the prescription for action laid the foundation for current strategies however, the chosen instruments for action gave, as yet, no indication that within three years very different actors would be called on to carry policy forward.

It is in the consideration of the most appropriate agencies for action that we can with hindsight see a puzzling inconsistency in the White Paper (puzzling, that is, until one remembers that this is the product of a Labour government). There would be a role for the private sector to play:

> Local authorities now need to stimulate investment by the private sector, by firms and by individuals, in industry, in commerce and in housing. The resources and energies of small and medium size firms are essential if real progress is to be made and the diversity and vitality, for so long characteristic of inner cities, is to be restored.

(Department of the Environment 1977e: 39)

Yet when the paper asserts that '*Local Authorities* are the natural agencies to tackle inner area problems' (Department of the Environment 1977e: 31) it does so not on the grounds that they would be best at stimulating and exploiting the necessary private sector investment (a question we shall examine subsequently) but rather on the grounds of their experience as *service providers* with their finger on the pulse of local needs and – a quite different issue – that they are democratically accountable. It was acknowledged that 'changes in approach by local and central government (would) be necessary', and that 'Local authorities with inner area problems will need to be more entrepreneurial in the attraction of industry and commerce' (Department of the Environment 1977e: 33). But this was in the context of a consideration and subsequent rejection of the possibility of using new town-style development corporations.

In short therefore, whilst the central strategy of the White Paper was the economic regeneration of the inner cities, the main instrument for its implementation was chosen (ostensibly at least) on the grounds of its experience in service delivery.[2] The government could have closed the coherence gap just by asserting that local authorities *were* the best instrument for stimulating and exploiting private sector investment. But would anyone have believed it?

THE FIRST TENTATIVE STEPS TOWARDS ENTERPRISE

Radical change changes our perceptions. At the time, the policy shifts consequent upon the White Paper seemed like a radical departure. In hindsight they look more like first faltering steps. The immediate policy implications were a new Inner Urban Areas Act in 1978 but, more importantly, a much increased budget (from £30m in 1977–8 to £125m in 1979–80 (Department of the Environment 1977e)), a new set of arrangements for the Urban Programme, and – because even the new level of funding appeared inadequate to the new task – the 'bending' of departments' main expenditure programmes and of the rate support grant to impact more discriminately on inner urban areas (see Edwards 1984: 598–9). The last of these had the air of a good wheeze that would make inner city expenditure levels more plausible. It would always be possible in the face of criticism about the inner city budget allocation to rejoin that of course that budget was but a small part of what the government would pump into the inner areas. A much larger (but thankfully indeterminate) amount would be 'bent' into the inner cities from main spending programmes and a rate support grant. It is a wheeze that governments have resorted to ever since. That the bending of service provision programmes did not sit easily with the new orthodoxy of stimulating private investment seems to have escaped notice. Anyway, the departments that were supposed to bend soon saw the idea off by keeping a straight tack, and whilst the rate support grant did bring additional benefit to the cities (but not of course directly to the *inner* cities) in the period to 1980, it thereafter veered off again towards the shires (Lansley 1979; Robson 1988: 98).

It was really in the revamped Urban Programme that the idea of stimulating private sector investment was to be accommodated, but while the apparatus of the programme was to change, the *method* of funding remained substantially unaltered. Thus, in place of a system by which in response to annual (and sometimes biannual) government circulars, local authorities and, through them, voluntary agencies, submitted bids for projects that would attract 75 per cent central government subsidy, there was now to be a priority listing of local authorities, ostensibly according to the degree of deprivation within them, and programme funds were to be concentrated to a greater degree on the more deprived areas. It wasn't fine targeting but it was a refinement of the old scattergun approach.

The details of the new arrangements have been extensively documented (Department of the Environment 1981a; Hall 1981; Lawless 1981; Home 1982; Whitting 1985; Rees and Lambert 1985; Sills *et al.* 1988) and we need not linger over them here, save to say that there were seven authorities (or areas, since they did not always coincide) in the 'first rank' of deprivation (the Partnership authorities), fifteen in the second rank (the Programme authorities), a further fourteen third rank 'Other Designated Districts' and then all remaining authorities which would be eligible for what now became known as the 'Traditional Urban Programme' or, less flatteringly, for the rump of resources left over when the other authorities had taken their cut. What is of more concern for our purposes is how, and what volume of resources were to be used within the new arrangements for the stimulation of private sector investment.

So far as the White Paper was concerned, the first tactic was to introduce an element of inner city bias into industrial and employment policies. The details were not spelled out but it appears that what was meant by an inner city bias was that regional industrial and employment policies should also have an intra-regional component, which in effect would have meant that they should be sufficiently finely tuned in spatial terms as to have dis-criminatory impact on inner city areas. There is no evidence however that at any time since 1977 have industrial and employment policies developed this degree of fine tuning – or anything like it.

The second strategy – and the one that was to be the genesis of most subsequent efforts to stimulate investment – was to use urban programme resources, particularly in the Partnership and Programme authorities, not as previously for preferentially funded service-provision projects, but rather to provide the incentives that would attract private investment to the inner cities and temporarily to prop up existing inner city businesses. In essence, the policy was, and ever since has been, despite numerous costume changes, to use public sector carrots to make inner city areas more competitive as industrial, commercial and retail sites. And it was this strategy as we shall see, whilst constituting only one of three spokes to urban programme funding in the years immediately following the White Paper, that gradually took both financial and presentational precedence over the others to become by the end of the 1980s the spearhead of inner city policy. (It was not a linear progression however. Four years after the White Paper, the Department of the Environment was still maintaining that 'the main role of the (new) Programme is to finance schemes which cannot easily slot into existing main programmes but are worthwhile in their own right' (Department of the Environment 1981a: 4). These were just the terms used to describe the purpose of the original Urban Programme and the (mainly) service provision projects funded under it. The air of residuality still seemed very much present, along with the need constantly to emphasise that the main work would be done elsewhere).

Though short on the details of how Urban Programme funding of partnership and programme authorities' inner area programmes (see Department of the Environment 1985) would in practice prevent inner city businesses from going under and – more importantly – attract new and relocating business that would otherwise have gone elsewhere, some of the ingredients were suggested. Many of these remain unchanged today, though other actors have taken over much of the responsibility. Thus, local authorities were to use their housing, planning and environmental powers to 'facilitate the growth of employment in inner areas'; they were to ensure that there were 'good industrial sites and premises available – with good communication'; and with certain additional powers they were to make loans to firms on commercial terms of up to 90 per cent for land purchase and for the erection or improvement of industrial buildings, establish industrial improvement areas, provide initial rent-free periods for factories and help out with the cost of site preparations. It is worth noting however that it is only in respect of the last two of these (rent 'holidays' and financial help with site preparations) that the White Paper referred to 'partnership areas' (they were it seems only to apply in these areas) and hence presumably to inner area programmes and the Urban Programme. All the other measures to be taken to attract investment were to be outwith the newly restructured Urban Programme. The apparent logic would seem to have been to shadow financial bending with the bending of such powers and regulations that local authorities had at their disposal as could and would have a more discriminatory impact on inner city areas. Once more, there is little evidence to suggest that the bending of powers has been any more successful than the bending of expenditures. Certainly, the story of inner city strategies throughout the 1980s has been the history of specific inner city policy rather than the bringing to bear on inner areas of main expenditure programmes and powers.

The new diagnosis, then, had been given a presentational high profile in the White Paper, and this was subsequently reiterated in a number of speeches by the then Secretary of State for the Environment, Peter Shore. He took the opportunity of a speech to the Royal Institution of Chartered Surveyors to press home the message that no pre-White Paper policies had addressed the problem of:

> loss of population and jobs from the inner city together with physical, social and economic decline. Our policy now is to halt that downward spiral; to strengthen the economic and social structures of the inner cities.
>
> (Department of the Environment 1978)

And yet for all the assertions of radical new policies to meet more fundamental problems, policy was in reality slow to follow the new path. Certainly there was the prioritisation of local authorities, and partnership and programme authorities had to draw up inner area programmes (to be funded at 75 per cent by central government as under the old Urban Programme) which were intended to be responses to local analyses of the particular requirements of the area. And an Inner Area Programme (IAP) was supposed to be just that – a coherent programme of action tailored to particular requirements. All too often however, IAPs consisted of a collection of discrete projects selected more on the criterion of giving all interested parties a crack of the whip than in the interests of strategic coherence. Notwithstanding that (in the partnership areas at least) there was a joint central–local government committee to oversee the collation of the programme and ensure its programmatic status, there was still (as ever) a multitude of interests to be satisfied (see Whitting 1985).

More significantly however, as we have noted, in the absence of any consistent financial or regulatory bending, such efforts as there were to promote the new strategy of economic regeneration were confined to the Urban Programme itself, and in particular to the IAPs of partnership and programme authorities. And these, quite apart from their (usually) un-programmatic nature, had other mandates to satisfy. By the time the social, environmental and housing requirements were allowed for, there was rela-tively little left in these early years for the stimulation of private sector investment. And as we shall see, whether because the private sector has an insatiable appetite for sweeteners or just because it takes a great deal of money to make many inner city areas at all competitive, the cost of economic regeneration would turn out to be greater than the funds available under the 'economic' head of the IAPs by a factor of hundreds. This we can say with hindsight. But in the years immediately following the White Paper, the strategy could only have looked plausible if a large part of it was to be fulfilled by activity outside the new Urban Programme. There must have been a belief that 'bending' would work; either that, or a monumental misconception of what economic regeneration would cost the public purse.

A COMMITMENT TO ENTERPRISE

The new arrangements were hardly in place before a general election brought a Conservative government to office, the ideological bent of which was very much in tune with the White Paper's approach – at least in terms of what the problem was and what needed to be done. On the question of the most appropriate instrument to pursue regeneration however, the new government would not be long in demonstrating its intention to change course fundamentally. What changed first – as would be expected – was the rhetoric. The inner cities, like everywhere else, were to be a part of the new revolution: enterprise had arrived. The first statement on the inner cities from the new Secretary of State for the Environment, Michael Heseltine, came four months after the election. However, its flavour had been rehearsed the previous year in a speech by Sir Geoffrey Howe to the Bow Group entitled *Liberating Free Enterprise: A New Experiment* (Howe 1978). Drawing on some ideas thrown out by Peter Hall in expansive mood, Sir Geoffrey outlined some of the elements of the enterprise zone idea – relaxed planning controls, disposal of land in public ownership, exemption from development land tax and possibly from local rates, absence of pay policies and price control and suspension of the Employment Protection Act. These ideas had been around for some time and in a variety of forms (such as Hong Kong-style 'freeports') but for the first time they were being brought to bear on the inner cities. Sir Geoffrey then went on to toy with some ideas about what sort of agency would be appropriate to administer these mini states; he didn't get far – but far enough to make it clear that local authorities would not be among them.

It is clear then that in this first flush of enthusiasm the identities of enterprise zones and urban development corporations had not yet been separated. There would be much hard graft to be put in to honing (and toning) down the enthusiasm into workable policies. But what was important was that there was an exciting new message to be got across: that nowhere – not least the inner cities – would escape the fresh winds of enterprise and initiative that would 'prime the pump of prosperity' and 'break through to a more dynamic future'. (The language of 'enterprise' mines a rich seam of metaphors.)

It is worth quoting at some length from Michael Heseltine's first statement as Secretary of State on the inner cities. The purpose of the statement (Department of the Environment 1979) was to announce a review of all inner city policies, but the opportunity was taken to put the stamp of the government's ideological credentials on the inner cities. From this document to the present day, the language of the enterprise culture has flavoured all the government's pronouncements on policies for inner urban areas. And their packaging has become glossier (some say in inverse relation to substance).

There was not a great deal for the document to say. The main substantive content was the announcement that the Secretary of State intended to take powers to enable the setting up of the first two Urban Development corporations (UDCs) in London's Docklands (then a Partnership area) and Merseyside Docklands. Other than that, the ostensible message was that existing components of the Urban Programme would be reviewed and that public expenditure restraints would prohibit any substantial growth in the inner city budget in the immediate future. The real messages of the statement were rooted in its language. The first was that the inner cities must be freed to allow enterprise to blossom. The second – a message that was to become more strident over the next decade – was that it was in large measure local government that they had to be freed from.

Having noted the concentration in the inner cities of those 'without choice – the elderly, the poor, the new (sic) immigrant communities (and) those whose only prospect of a home was on a municipal estate' (Department of the Environment 1979: 1), the statement asserts that:

> we want to make it possible for growth and prosperity to return to the inner cities again. The objectives are to make our inner cities places where people want to live and work, and where *the private investor is prepared to put his money.*
>
> (Department of the Environment 1979: 1, emphasis added)

And again, there must be a place in the inner cities 'for individual initiative and enterprise to get on the move . . .'.

The statement ends with Mr Heseltine's vision and creed for the inner cities:

> I would like to see inner cities once again be full of hustle and bustle on a human scale, varied, alive, above all places where people are free to develop and to succeed.
>
> (Department of the Environment 1979: 3)

Of course, we should not put too much store by this sort of thing; it was the ideological icing for a cake that had not yet been baked. But even by the standards of inner city policies, it was all rather vacuous. *Somehow* enterprise was going to create, from decayed areas with concentrations of the poor and dependent, communities of human-scale hustle and bustle alive with the freedom to succeed. Was this to be the renaissance of the urban craft workshop economy?

As for the role of the public sector (for which, in this context, we may read 'local government'), its demotion at this stage was muted, but the first markers were being put down: 'The public sector has a role to play. . .but we should not exaggerate it as I believe the previous government did.' And on the topic of the composition of partnership and programme authorities' inner area programmes, the Secretary of State said, 'we shall certainly wish to ensure that the balance of the programmes is influenced by people employed other than in the public sector' (Department of the Environment 1979: 2).

The two themes that would (and continue to) inform inner city policies were therefore established at a very early date. It seemed, in 1979, to be in large measure a continuation of the Labour government's policies (apart from pressing ahead with the UDCs – something that Labour had only dallied with) but as the promotion of enterprise and the exclusion of local government became increasingly dominant, so it became clear that this was to be a radical departure rather than a slight alteration of course.

When the review of inner city policies was published in 1981 it was, in retrospect, a modest document, proposing little significant change. Most importantly, there was to be a further increase in urban programmes allocation to £215m (from £93m in 1978–9 and £202m in 1980–1). Other than that, the establishment of the two UDCs was confirmed and the partnership and programme arrangements and designated authorities would remain unchanged. The commitment to main programme 'bending', however, was qualified and less than 'firm'. (Indeed, so profligate was the government's use of the adjective at this time that any commitment that wasn't 'firm' could be considered to be positively flaccid.) Thus on bending, the Secretary of State said:

> Allocations under main programme, which, despite reductions remain the largest components of public investment in inner cities, will continue *where possible* to take into account their needs.
>
> (Department of the Environment 1981b: 2)

Such other measures as were proposed were designed to promote the new orthodoxies – enterprise, efficiency, and the demotion of local government. The partnership and programme authorities were to simplify their inner area programme (IAP) procedures and make them more efficient. 'Effective consultation' with local industry and commerce in preparing the IAPs would become a *prior condition* of receipt of grant. And there would be a shift in the schemes funded under the Urban Programme towards those that 'strengthened local economies'.

1981: LAYING THE GROUNDWORK

In other respects, 1981 turned out to be an eventful year for the inner cities. It saw the establishment of the first two urban development corporations, the first nine enterprise zones (which were announced by the Chancellor of the Exchequer in his 1980 budget and which, until the repackaging of inner city policies in the two *Action for Cities* brochures in 1987 and 1988 (Department of the Environment 1987, Cabinet Office 1988), the Department of the Environment claimed were not a part of inner city policy (Department of the Environment 1982a: 10, para II, 23)), a number of local enterprise agencies and the Financial Institutions Group in Merseyside. When these are added to the reorientation of Urban Programme resources away from social and environmental projects and towards economic ones, and from revenue to capital expenditure, we can see that the new orthodoxy was beginning to inform policy in a more concrete way. It would be wrong to view the events of 1981 as part of a concerted and coherent package however. The drift of all these separate items was in the same direction – an emphasis on the role of the private sector, the leverage of private sector funds and the abbreviation of the local government role – but their roots were in diverse places. The idea of enterprise zones and urban agencies (what became the urban development corporations) had been around for some time as we have noted, and the shift in Urban Programme resources was a direct outcome of the policy review. The civil disturbances also accounted for a spate of new ideas and some reappraisal of policy, although their direct influence on new policy generation has not, with the benefit of hindsight, been as extensive as has sometimes been claimed. There is no doubt that at the time however, they caused a stir in policy circles. In the paper that he wrote for the Cabinet at the time, *It Took a Riot*, Heseltine made a number of specific proposals requiring 'substantial additional public resources' to cope with extremes of need in the inner city areas. These proposals were not adopted; they were referred to a sub-committee and never reached full Cabinet (see Hennessy 1989: 705–8). But what survived, and (unlike proposals for more public expenditure) won the Prime Minister's support, were suggestions for closer involvement of business and industry in the revival of the inner cities: as it was subsequently expressed, the return of the (so-called) City Fathers – local businessmen who had once provided the social and economic core of local urban communities.

Heseltine's own philosophy was summed up in *Where There's a Will*:

that leadership awakens a response; that the public and private sectors work best in partnership; and that British capitalists can show a well-developed sense of public duty.

(Heseltine 1987)

Only the Financial Institutions Group (FIG), that now legendary charabanc full of financiers, with Mr Heseltine as tour courier, had any direct provenance in the civil disturbances of 1981 however. This was an act of 'faith in the City', the first real test for enterprise. It is doubtful that Mrs Thatcher approved – she wanted, as an article of her faith – that the government be seen *not* to respond to the riots, but Mr Heseltine saw the opportunity to demonstrate that the engine of enterprise was the right instrument to turn the inner cities around. And it was probably only the overheated post-riot atmosphere when everyone was peddling their own patent solution that induced twenty-six financiers to take a bus ride round inner Liverpool.

We shall dwell briefly on the FIG initiative here because it came and went within twelve months and because some of its recommendations were to influence future strategies. Its passage across the inner cities stage was a fleeting one (unlike some other initiatives canvassed here, an examination of which forms the substance of subsequent chapters) but its legacy is out of proportion to the length of its life. The coach trip was a gesture, of course; the purpose was to get some representatives of banks, building societies, insurance companies and pension funds to join common purpose with the government to demonstrate the influence of enterprise. It was in a way a common affirmation by government and private finance of their common belief in a new culture. And the imagery was powerful: enterprise to the rescue where a plodding and divided local government had allowed such dreadful things to happen. Mr Heseltine got what he wanted – the coach party agreed to second a group of middle managers from their institutions for one year who, with civil servants from the department, would make up the FIG. The objective of the group was: 'the development of new approaches and ideas for securing urban regeneration, including greater involvement of financial institutions and the private sector generally' (House of Commons Environment Committee 1982–3: 506). The results of their year's deliberations came in both tangible and less tangible forms, according to the Department of the Environment's own assessment. The tangible output was a list of recommendations for private sector involvement in urban regeneration.

The less tangible benefits were outlined in a memorandum from the Department of the Environment to the House of Commons Environment Committee taking evidence on the problems of management of urban renewal during its 1982–3 session. They related to the educative effects of the exercise both for the private sector managers (and their institutions) and the civil servants. The financial institutions, argued the memorandum, were exposed by the exercise 'to the idea of working together with the Government, and to urban problems hitherto regarded as exclusively for the public sector' (House of Commons Environment Committee 1982–3, Minutes of Evidence: 507, para 33).

In the other direction, the memorandum continued:

> Civil servants (had) worked for a year very closely with people from the major financial institutions who in most cases had remained based in those institutions and had a direct link to top management. Thus, the Department was given an unprecedented opportunity to see how the institutions reacted to proposals affecting them, and what their working methods, attitudes and capabilities were; and. . .how managers with a training in various private sector disciplines *approached social or policy problems*. In the context of an overall policy aimed at increasing private sector involvement on urban questions, the exercise was very useful.
>
> (House of Commons Environment Committee 1982–3, Minutes of
> Evidence: 507, para 34, emphasis added)

How much of this was dressing for the Committee's sake and how much a substantive learning process, is impossible to say. Movement between policy areas is fairly frequent in the middle and senior civil service and whether there would be any lasting effects from exposure to the private sector would depend in large measure on the transmissibility of the 'new' culture from one individual to another. On the face of it, it would seem that the culture of privatism would be hard pressed to have much impact on the culture of Whitehall. The latter we know is a strong integrating force in the Whitehall village (see for example Heclo and Wildavsky 1974; Edwards 1981; Williams 1988) and a powerful component of it is its patrician attitude to the private sector and anything that whiffs of trade. And the fact that the chaps at the Department of Trade and Industry had been rubbing shoulders with the private sector for a number of years without obvious sign of serious deterioration in their psyches was perhaps a tribute to the resilience of the Whitehall culture.

According to one commentator, however, the blending worked: 'with regulars and irregulars having a great deal to teach and to learn from each other' (Hennessy 1989: 710). Hennessy further quotes one of the irregulars drafted in from consultants Peat Marwick McLintock:

> It was a very pioneering atmosphere in the Department of the Environment Inner Cities Directorate in 1982. The policy was being executed by ministers and their officials and by us private sector secondees with

great enthusiasm. We were all charting very new ground. It hadn't really been done before.

(Howard Mallinson as quoted in Hennessy 1989: 710)

Notwithstanding Hennessy's useful account, the meeting and merging of the privatism culture and the culture of Whitehall and its effect on policy and policy output is largely uncharted territory especially in so far as recent inner city policies are concerned. Indeed, as has been argued elsewhere (Edwards 1981), it is extremely difficult to identify policy outputs that have been influenced and changed by the particular cultural milieu within which they are developed; but that the Whitehall culture has been and continues to be a potent force in policy has been attested to by a number of commentators (see, for example, Metcalfe and Richards 1987; Williams 1988).

For the moment, it is only possible to speculate on whether the FIG experience left a flavour (or a taint) of privatism in the Whitehall culture. Certainly, the department was anxious to give the impression that this had been a constructive learning exercise, and there is evidence elsewhere to suggest that incoming ministers' views of civil servants were only marginally warmer than their views of local authorities and, charged with the spirit of enterprise, they would brook no hindrance from them. On the other hand, other than doing their ministers' bidding, it seems unlikely that the FIG initiative would have made any lasting impact on the *ways* in which policy was made. However, this story remains yet to be told.

Another development in 1981 that has so far stayed the course is Business in the Community (BiC). This was established in 1981 after a Conference at Sunningdale organised by the DoE and chaired by the then Minister for Local Government, Tom King. One of the key objectives of BiC has been to establish Local Enterprise Agencies (LENTAs) in all major cities. Over 300 now exist; they are collaborations between public and private sectors led by local business, providing business counselling and other forms of training and support services, linked with existing statutory provision. Business in the Community is not a component of the government's inner city policy, but it is often cited in departmental brochures as an example of the efficacy of the private sector in helping to alleviate social problems (see, for example, House of Commons Environment Committee 1982–3: 510–11), and its line of approach is one of the major recommendations of the CBI's review of inner city action, *Initiatives Beyond Charity* (1988). The basis thesis of this influential report was that:

cities will. . .have to spring from sound economic development, driven by private sector investment decisions taken on the basis of the commercial returns available, not from a sense of charity.

(Confederation of British Industry 1988: 9)

There is an aura of 'corporate social responsibility' around BiC but the bottom line is corporate self-interest: this is the Chief Executive of American Express describing his company's membership: 'Call it enlightened self-interest. Call it altruism. I call it common business sense. However you look at it, it's good business to be a community player' (Vulliamy 1988). And another BiC publication urges private enterprise to invest in the inner cities on the grounds that:

> Strife and decay in the inner cities and associated threats to property and public safety carry a high political risk – neglect will eventually impose a high cost on the whole business community.
>
> (BiC undated, as quoted in Barnekov *et al.* 1989: 207)

The implication of such attitudes of course is that the private sector will only invest in the inner cities so long as there is a coincidence of interests. And membership of, and financial contribution to, the BiC club is, for many companies, probably of the same degree of significance – and for largely the same reasons as their contributions to the Conservative Party funds – an insurance premium.

A less structured arrangement but one with the same broad purposes arose in the early 1980s in the form of local groupings of senior businessmen and specialists from the commercial sector: chambers of commerce were seen as particularly promising vehicles for such an approach. These groups were (and are) intended to fill the vacuum of leadership left by the remoteness of central government and the inadequacies of local political leadership. Local business leaders are encouraged to 'come out' as part of the process of filling this gap: their public commitment will have value as a catalyst and also for public relations purposes. An example of this approach is The Newcastle Initiatives (TNI); the major evidence of success being achieved is the completion of a major 'flagship' development scheme, the cranes on the horizons signifying Action (a word for which BiC has a particular fondness).

Then there is British Urban Development (BUD), the purpose of which again is to promote private sector development in the inner cities. BUD is however essentially a consortium of developers which concentrates its work particularly on UDCs and by so doing can build up an expertise and specialised knowledge which give it more of the air of a trade association.

Variants of these techniques and arrangements underpin the new approach adopted more recently by central government to training – the creation of local business-led Training and Enterprise Councils (TECs) to take over the main responsibilities of the former Training Agency (the Manpower Services Commission); and in the education field, the City Technology Colleges (CTCs), to be established with dowries from local employers to provide intensive programmes of technical education outside the mainstream of the state system. (Although these are not intended to be located specifically within the inner cities, they have been promoted as part of inner city policy.)

There is an area of uncertainty that most of these arrangements generate – and one that it is our purpose to examine in subsequent chapters. It relates to the circumstances in which the private sector is prepared to invest in the inner cities and what the limits of those circumstances are.

1981–90: ENTERPRISE THE MEANS – AND SOMETIMES THE END

Between 1981 and 1990 a number of new initiatives were begun, all emphasising in some degree an enhanced role for the private sector in urban regeneration. Perhaps more significantly however, the enterprise rhetoric became both stronger and increasingly attached, as the decade progressed, to the urban development corporations which, numbering ten by the end of the decade, were promoted as the spearhead of the government's efforts.

Other than the Financial Institutions Group and Business in the Community, there were eight important policy developments during the 1980s. Some of these will receive more extensive treatment in subsequent chapters and we need only at this stage identify their place and role in the growing ascendancy of the private sector in inner city regeneration. Because they constitute the main (though, as we have noted, by no means the complete) body of policy development during the decade, they are listed below for ease of reference:

- Urban Development Grants (1982)
- A special inner-city priority category for Derelict Land Grant (1982/82)
- Garden Festivals (the first in 1984)
- City Action Teams (the first eight in 1985)
- Task Forces (1986/87)
- Urban Regeneration Grant (1987)
- City Grant (1988)
- Urban Development Corporations (a further eight in 1987–8)

Urban Development Grant

Based on the American Urban Development Action Grant (see Barnekov *et al.* 1989: 72–4, 79–86), Urban Development Grant is the only component of inner cities policy that is explicitly acknowledged to have provenance in an American programme (Department of the Environment 1982b: ii), though Barnekov *et al.* claim that its genesis went further back than the deliberations of the Financial Institutions Group to which credit is usually given. Urban Development Grant was a part of the Urban Programme but, more than any other part, its singular purpose was to involve the private sector. In essence, it was a central government grant available *only* for capital expenditure on development projects that had been designed collaboratively between local authorities and the private sector. A substantial private sector input was a *sine qua non*, and a 'vital ingredient' of schemes was that they should provide more employment opportunities for inner city residents (see Department of the Environment 1983).

It is noteworthy that of the two elements to the increasing involvement of enterprise in inner city polices, UDG promoted only one. At this stage (1982), there was to be more private sector involvement (financially and otherwise) but the demotion of local authorities had not yet begun. Proposals for grant-aided schemes could only be submitted by local authorities (having been worked up jointly with private sector institutions), a system of application that was consistent with the other parts of the Urban Programme. In fact, local authorities were not to be cut out of UDG until it was merged with Urban Regeneration Grant and a part of the Derelict Land Grant in 1988.

The aims of UDG as set out in the Guidance Notes were:

> to act as a stimulus to the *economic* regeneration of our urban areas. . .real economic growth and development cannot be sustained without the close involvement of the private sector. U.D.G. is intended to sharpen the incentives to the private sector . . .
>
> (Department of the Environment 1982b: i, emphasis added)

But what in particular the scheme inherited from the American UDAG programme was the idea of 'leverage' – a term that was to become increasingly familiar in the language of inner city policy during the remainder of the decade. In the words of the Guidance Notes again:

> U.D.G. is designed to lever significant private sector investment into the inner cities, providing *the minimum public sector contribution* necessary to enable development projects which might not otherwise go ahead to do so.
>
> (Department of the Environment 1982b: ii, emphasis added)

This idea of a minimum public sector contribution necessary to lever as much private sector investment as possible was later to be formalised as the 'gearing ratio' – a measure that Urban Development Corporations would come to adopt as the gauge of their virility.

Before we leave UDG, it is worth noting that although they pushed the involvement of the private sector in public policy up a notch or two, their introduction was not marked by any overall increase in funds for the inner cities. The initial allocation for UDG was £70m which turned out to be an earmarked slice of funds already allocated to the Urban Programme.

Derelict Land Grant

The idea of a public: private investment ratio was given explicit recognition a year later when the Secretary of State for the Environment, Mr Tom King, announced the redesigned Derelict Land Grant (it was not yet a gearing ratio). Once again, the DLG was introduced as a measure by which public funds would be used to 'attract substantially greater amounts of private investment'. On this occasion, Mr King was able to provide some specifics:

> I am today approving £30 million of derelict land grant for 46 projects that will lead to £200 million of additional private sector investment. . . an impressive ratio of one to six of public to private funds.
>
> (House of Commons 1983: col. 159)

There is no record of whether the £200m materialised in the areas, but subsequent experience of gearing ratio calculations suggests that they are – to put it charitably – fairly flexible.

Garden Festivals

The next chronological developments in our story were the Garden Festivals, the first of which was organised by the nascent Merseyside Development Corporation and held in Liverpool in 1984 (Hansard, House of Commons 1984: col. 118). Subsequent festivals were held in Stoke, Gateshead and Ebbw Vale (Department of the Environment 1987: paras 16–19; Department of the Environment 1988a: 6; Department of the Environment 1990a: 34). However, these add little to our story of the growing hegemony of the private sector in inner city policy except that recent ones have not turned out to be the financial successes that were anticipated.

City Action Teams

The first five City Action Teams (CATs) were created in 1985 and a further three were subsequently added. Their significance for our account lies in the fact that they were the first attempt at co-ordinating the roles of the growing number of agencies involved in inner city regeneration. No doubt the increasingly prominent part played by the private sector had served further to confuse an already complex plot, with too many actors appearing either to be playing the same roles or to be participating in a different play altogether. It seems reasonable to assume therefore that not the least part of the function of CATs was to ease the way for enterprise through the maze of local and central government agencies already at work in the partnership areas (Department of the Environment, Department of Trade and Industry and Department of Employment 1985).

Task Forces

Eight Task Forces were announced in 1986 and a further eight in 1987. Since then, some have closed down 'having done their job' and others have opened, but the total number at any one time has remained at sixteen. The distinctive features of task forces are that they are highly targeted – focusing on quite small areas with around 30,000 population, they are intended to have a bias towards areas of ethnic minority concentration, and to be relatively short-lived (the 'quick fixes' of inner city policy). Their aims, as initially stated by Mr Kenneth Clarke, then Paymaster General and responsible in the House for Employment matters, were to improve job and business prospects in the targeted areas using small amounts of seed money (approximately £1 million per Task Force) to lever more resources from the private sector, main government spending programmes, charities and trusts (House of Commons: Hansard 1986). There were (and are) two prongs therefore to the Task Force purpose: firstly to stimulate local business and hence strengthen local economies, and secondly to prepare local residents to be more competitive in the job market by means of skills training and, where possible, more customised training (Department of Trade and Industry 1989). Which of these two was to have precedence may be judged from the fact that when Mr Clarke and his senior, Lord Young, were moved to the Department of Trade and Industry in the post-election shuffle of 1987, the Task Forces went with them.

Despite the government's desire not to be seen to be moved by urban violence, there can be no other adequate explanation for the creation of the Task Forces than the civil unrest that had preceded their announcement. And both St Pauls in Bristol and Handsworth in Birmingham, which were among the first eight Task Forces to be created, had been the scenes of civil disturbance involving large numbers of young people from ethnic minorities. Their aims were not fundamentally different (other than in the precision of their targeting and their focus on ethnic minorities) from those of a number of other initiatives such as the urban development corporations, the Enterprise Zones and, in particular the inner area programmes of the Urban Programme, with which, in a number of instances, they overlapped geographically.

But if, as seems reasonable to assume, their implicit purpose was to reduce the likelihood of repeated civil unrest, the 'solution' differed in no significant way from what had by now become the panacea for most social ills – the nurturing of enterprise. This is how Mr Clarke put it when announcing the task forces:

> We shall seek to stimulate enterprise and provide a stronger base for the local economy. We shall give special attention to the problems of young people from ethnic minorities where they are particularly disadvantaged.
> (Clarke 1988)

No explicit connection was made between urban unrest, ethnic minorities and the new Task Forces, but the timing of the announcement and the juxtaposition of its contents leave little doubt.

Urban Regeneration Grant

Until 1986 (and excepting the UDCs) only one prong of the enterprise strategy had been developed – the promotion of private sector investment. There had been no serious attempts positively to implement the second arm – the diminution of the role of the public sector in general but local government in particular. The first explicit move in this direction came with the introduction of Urban Regeneration Grant (URG) which was designed to complement Urban Development Grant. Provision for URG was made in the Housing and Planning Act of 1986 and grant became operative in April the following year. Its signal feature was that it was payable directly to private developers without having to pass through local authorities and without the proposed development having to receive local authority approval. For the first time therefore, a component of inner city policy was cutting local authorities out of the financial process. Indeed, it was excluding them from participation in the development. There were other notable aspects to URG: it allowed the Department of the Environment to offer grant assistance outside areas designated under the Inner Urban Areas Act 1978, and it enabled whole-site improvement rather than assistance with the renewal of individual buildings (see Barnekov *et al.* 1989: 190); but without doubt, its longer-term significance lay in the exclusion of local authorities. Indeed, this singular feature was extended in March 1988 when URG was merged with UDG and part of the DLG into the new City Grant, *all* assistance under which was to be paid directly to private developers.

City Grant

The new City Grant was designed to support capital development projects undertaken by the private sector where return on investment would otherwise be marginal (Department of the Environment 1988b). Thus, by combining three development grants into one, the government was quickly able to extend the role of the private sector and to exclude local government from participating in another component of inner city policies. And, as with all other schemes designed to attract private sector investment, the success of City Grant was to be measured in terms of its gearing ratio.

Urban Development Corporations

The drive to put private enterprise at the forefront of inner city regeneration gained momentum rapidly in 1987 and 1988 with the creation of eight new Urban Development Corporations, their promotion as the spearhead of inner city policies, and the high-profile publicity launch of *Action for Cities*.

The government has described UDCs as 'single minded agencies (able) to unlock the full potential of inner city areas' (Department of the Environment 1990a: 10). The message, none too subtle, is that local authorities are neither. They have also been described as the 'flagships' of the enterprise-driven approach to the redevelopment of the inner city, and this is an accurate perception in so far as they embody the aspirations of the first Secretary of State for the Environment in the Conservative Government elected in 1979. Michael Heseltine has described how he confronted his Permanent Secretary, Sir John Garlick, with a series of policy proposals for immediate consideration, of which development corporations in the inner cities was high on the list (Heseltine 1987). This proposal was based on Heseltine's perception of the (relative) failure of the public-sector-driven policies of his Labour predecessor, Peter Shore, and the sense of an opportunity that existed, in physical form in the derelict Docklands area and structurally in the creation of new bodies that would be empowered to take decisive action out with the constraints of the planning system and over-lapping tiers of local government with conflicting objectives. It was also an opportunity to demonstrate the effectiveness of the private sector.

Urban Development Corporations were born of this perception. The legislation that enabled them to be established, the Local Government Planning and Land Act, 1980, pre-empted the danger of lengthy public enquiries by giving the Secretary of State power to establish UDCs if, in his opinion, it is 'expedient in the national interest to do so'. The aim of a UDC is to secure the regeneration of the area designated, chiefly in terms of the physical renewal of land and buildings. After taking advice, the Secretary of State defines the area and appoints a Board to run the UDC. The expectation is that the Board will be composed primarily of representatives of business interests, although it is customary to offer seats to members of local authorities within whose area the UDC will be operating. The Board in turn appoints the Chief Executive and a range of other officers – usually with responsibilities for planning, marketing and public relations. The expectation has been that a substantial number of executive tasks will be put out to contract with outside consultants, so that the size of staff employed will remain relatively small.

The powers of the UDC are very substantial. It can:

- grant planning permission for developments in its area;
- acquire, hold, manage and dispose of land in its area (it can either use Compulsory Purchase orders to acquire land or ask the Secretary of State to vest public sector land to it);
- provide water, electricity, gas, sewerage and other services;
- provide various forms of grants and financial aid to developers.

UDCs also have reserve powers to engage in other forms of activity in general support of the objective of regeneration.

These activities are supported by central government grants provided on an annual basis from the DoE's urban block allocation. In addition, UDCs may raise funds through loans to support commercially viable projects. The Secretary of State's control is exercised through the setting of an annual External Finance Limit (EFL) covering grants and loans made by the UDC – although receipts from land sales may also be used as a top-up which does not count against the EFL. In addition, the Secretary of State requires the UDC to produce an annual Corporate Plan and to submit individual projects for departmental approval.

The funds obtained in this way from public sources are of course to be used to 'lever' private sector investment and development into the area. In this way, the right environment for economic regeneration is created. Unlike the new town development corporations on which Michael Heseltine based the original concept, the UDC is not primarily intended to function as an executive agency that delivers services. Rather, it facilitates activity by other agencies, principally those from the private sector. These activities focus explicitly on physical redevelopment. As Robin Butler, the civil servant responsible for the programme, told the House of Commons Employment Committee in 1988, Urban Development Corporations 'are about regeneration and, indeed, about physical regeneration of their areas, and this is where the primary thrust of their activity is concerned' (Stoker 1989: 164). Once this regeneration has been achieved the UDC's function is complete and it can be wound up – the expectation being that this will be secured within ten to fifteen years from declaration (National Audit Office 1988; House of Commons Employment Committee 1988a; Stoker 1989).

The UDCs have been declared in three distinct phases. The first, as we have noted, was in 1981, when the LDDC and Merseyside DC were established. In his account of the process, Heseltine comments that his proposals had a 'rough ride' in Cabinet. Apparently, they offended against the new government's commitment to the reduction of quangos; perhaps more important, 'the Treasury perceived a wide opening for additional public expenditure'. But the Prime Minister 'overruled objections, sharing my view that the deadhand of Socialism should be lifted' and that 'along the Thames and the Mersey, the sinews to recreate the environment, the opportunities and incentives for reconstruction that had been so unhappily destroyed' should now be provided (Heseltine 1987: 136). This linkage is deceptive, however, because the two initial UDCs were very different in character and circumstances. This emerged clearly in the diverse experience of the two areas after declaration. (We shall pursue the case of the London Docklands in more detail in Chapter 6 of this volume.)

There was a long gap between the establishment of LDDC and MDC and further designations. The years 1987–9 however witnessed a large increase in the government's promotion of enterprise and a very significant component of this was the designation of eight new UDCs in England and one in Wales. Between February and May 1987 Trafford Park, Teesside, Tyne and Wear and Black Country UDCs were created along with Cardiff (the only UDC in Wales), and in December of the same year a further three smaller UDCs were announced for Bristol, Leeds and Central Manchester. The eighth English corporation – in Sheffield – was announced in March 1988. Between them, the ten British corporations are responsible for some 40,000 acres of land (Department of the Environment 1990b: 8) and total grants-in-aid to them from the Department of the Environment in 1988–9 stood at £234 million, representing 40.6 per cent of all central government expenditure on inner cities programmes, that is, UDCs, City Grant, the Urban Programme, Enterprise Zones and land registers (Department of the Environment 1990a: 6). Planned expenditure on UDCs and the proportion of total inner cities expenditure that goes to them increased in 1990–1 and will decline thereafter to 1993 (Department of the Environment 1990a: 6).

What we therefore find in the closing years of the 1980s is the use of the UDC strategy, quiescent since 1981, to give substance to the growing conviction that enterprise, and only enterprise, could do the job. Local authorities (but especially Labour-controlled ones) were a hindrance. (Whether the job they could do was the one that needed doing is a question to which we devote our attentions in subsequent chapters.) And the message was made explicit on a number of occasions. Of UDCs, the government's *Action for Cities* brochure claimed:

> Their special executive powers enable them to cut through red tape and press on with action. They take decisions on the use of land and they

have the financial means to clear dereliction and get development under way. They are a prime example of the government's determination to take effective action to encourage business and new investment.

(Cabinet Office 1988: 4)

'Cutting through', 'pressing on', 'determination' and '*effective* action' (never 'action') are all hallmarks of the enterprise culture. The same document maintains that UDCs 'are the most important attack ever made on urban decay. They are already transforming inner cities' (Cabinet Office 1988: 12), and the next brochure made it quite explicit that they 'are at the forefront of the government's drive to revitalise the inner cities' (Department of the Environment 1989a: 12). (Not only does your action have to be 'effective' in the enterprise culture, it has to be driven as well.)

The announcement of the last urban development corporation in the Don Valley of Sheffield was made at the *Action for Cities* publicity occasion on 7 March 1988 and, apart from an increase in the area of the Merseyside Development Corporation, it was the only announcement of substance at this strange event. What had been intended as a White Paper to give substance to Mrs Thatcher's election night rallying call was found on examination to have very little substance at all. It fell to the advertising agency Young and Rubicam to turn a potential embarrassment into a symbol of drive and purpose – something to be waved aloft by ministers and their leader. This was to be inner city policy designer style; never mind the contents, look at the pretty packaging. It is described in the Prime Minister's foreword as an 'action document' describing what 'adds up to a £3,000 million major attack' (the first and only time that figure has been used). But the main purpose of *Action for Cities* (not to be confused with a similar document with the same title issued the previous year jointly by a number of departments) is to convey the message of enterprise:

'The government has created a climate which supports enterprise and has set about removing obstacles in the way of inner city recovery.

(Cabinet Office 1988: Foreword)

The country is rediscovering enterprise and resourcefulness. There is a new national self-confidence.

(Cabinet Office 1988: 3)

In similar vein, during the press conference, Mr Kenneth Clarke, then inner cities co-ordinator, maintained:

We believe that we can persuade yet more businessmen that it is a sensible commercial activity for a successful company to play a leading role in regenerating cities which are their trading base.

(Clarke 1988)

And Mr Nicholas Ridley, then at Environment, denied that he wanted to cut out local authorities, but merely to 'get rid of obstacles so that investors can invest'.

Action for Cities (1988) is silent on health or social services provision, says nothing about education (other than job training) and does not mention welfare benefits. The words poverty, deprivation and inequity are absent. It is as if they no longer existed; what was wanting was enterprise, and once it had been rekindled it would do the job – and presumably the whole job. And as if to demonstrate that it was putting its money where its mouth was, the government included figures in *Action for Cities* that showed that the proportion of total inner cities expenditure that went on assisting private investment (as opposed to going to social and community projects) increased from 66 per cent in 1979–80 to 77 per cent in 1983–4 and 83 per cent in 1988–9. Ten months after the press conference however, the White Paper on government expenditure plans for 1989–90 showed inner city spending would be cut by £17 million in 1989–90 and by £30 million by 1992.[2]

Of course, if the enterprise culture were really to take hold, there would be little need for any public expenditure on the inner cities.

NOTES

1   There are exceptions to every generalisation; Harvey in the USA and Cullingworth in Britain were both, from different perspectives, able to write about the urban core in a broader framework that enabled them at least to encroach on the reasons for central urban decay (see Harvey 1973; Cullingworth 1973).

2   These projections turned out to be more than usually erratic. At least, they are difficult to square with the figures in the Department of the Environment Annual Report for 1992 which show *increases* in expenditure for both 1989–90 and 1990–91 but an estimated downturn in 1991–92 (see Table 2.1).

Table 2.1 Central government expenditure on inner cities: England

£ million

	1986/87	1987/88	1988/89	1989/90	1990/91	1991/92
Urban Programme	236.8	245.6	224.3	222.7	225.8	242.4
City Grants	23.9	26.8	27.8	39.1	45.4	55.5
Derelict Land	78.1	76.5	67.8	54.0	61.7	75.6
Urban Development Corporations	89.3	133.5	234.4	436.0	553.6	501.5
City Action Teams	–	–	–	4.0	7.7	8.1
Other	14.2	7.9	8.3	7.0	–2.0	0.8
Total	442.4	490.3	562.6	762.8	892.2	883.8

Note: Estimates
Source: Department of the Environment Annual Report, 1992

3 Is inner city policy about urban deprivation?

The logic of the process whereby enterprise investment and the promulgation of an enterprise culture will reduce deprivation (whatever that turns out to be) has never been fully specified either by responsible government departments (least of all by them) or by academic and other commentators. In this and Chapter 4 we shall try to spell out at least some of the ways in which the process might work. This has to be to some extent speculative however, because it must be remembered that there is no evidence that the wide range of policies now available has been developed on the foundation of a clear understanding of how they would make an impact. That is why we have to say that when we come to consider the detail of how the regenerative process operates, we have to think in terms of how it *might* work. We are simply wanting of any detailed specification of how it *will* work or even of how it is *intended* to work. The danger in this of course is that we may be accused of imputing aims and intentions to policies that they were never meant to carry and in so doing will write failure into our evaluation. There is substance in this argument and it deserves a reply. There are, as we shall see later, more than thirty policies or programmes that in varying degrees may be said to be concerned with the inner cities, and between them they will carry a variety of aims.

It is the view of the Department of the Environment and other interested departments that these programmes are complementary and that they are all aimed at different parts of the problem. The enterprise solution therefore (so the argument goes) is but one of a number, that it is not intended to have an impact on all aspects of the inner city problem, and that there are a number of other programmes, not focused around economic regeneration, which will do the job that enterprise cannot (and was never intended to) do. The argument is less than compelling however, mainly for the reasons we outlined in Chapter 2. All recent publications on inner city policy have emphasised strongly and repeatedly that the government is wedded to the enterprise solution and that the use of the private sector to effect economic regeneration is their cardinal strategy for dealing with the inner cities. Indeed, if we extract those programmes dedicated to this strategy (including the Urban Programme within which the emphasis is now on capital projects and projects to promote economic growth) then there is little that is left. If the enterprise strategy will not alleviate deprivation, in all its manifestations, then there is little else on the books at present that will.

In order to give emphasis to the arguments outlined above, we shall begin our analysis by trawling a number of recent (and some less recent) statements of the aims of inner city policies from government publications (which we must take to be reasonably authoritative sources). Having established at least the flavour of the intentions of policy, we shall be in a position to compare these with the Department of the Environment's own formulation of the nature of deprivation and the inner city problem more generally. This, however, will turn out to be less than comprehensive and will need to be filled out in order to provide a more accurate picture of the range of manifestations of deprivation. And it is this composite list of the components of deprivation that we shall use in our attempt in Chapter 4 to articulate the logic of how enterprise may have an impact on deprivation. The effectiveness of inner city policies (or those of them – the majority – that have economic regeneration as their strategy) will also depend however on the manner of their implementation and, in particular, their use of area designations as we noted in Chapter 1. When we come to examine the logic of the enterprise culture therefore in Chapter 4, we will consider in more detail the potential effectiveness of the area approach in alleviating deprivation and – a related question – the appropriateness of trying to 'reverse history'.

THE AIMS OF INNER CITY POLICIES

The broad direction of inner city policies was established by the 1977 White Paper. A number of variations have been written on the theme since then; there have been presentational modifications; what was muted then has become more strident now, and the motif of enterprise has become insistent.

Other than the 'bending' of main programme expenditures and rate support grant (neither of which, as we have already noted, came to fruition) the drafters of the 1977 White Paper had some variation of the original Urban Programme in mind when they articulated the 'underlying aims' of future inner cities policy. And although the enterprise solution had not yet come to the fore (there were to be two more years of Labour government), the idea of economic regeneration was planted, but was still to be effected by a revised Urban Programme. These underlying aims were:

a) strengthening the economies of the inner areas and the prospects of their residents;

b) improving the physical fabric of the inner areas and making their environment more attractive;

c) alleviating social problems;

d) securing a new balance between the inner areas and the rest of the city region in terms of populations and jobs.

(Department of the Environment 1977e, para 26)

It is worth emphasising that these were the aims of inner city policy in general; they were drafted with the Urban Programme in mind but the Urban Programme would *be* inner city policy for at least the next four years.

The first three of these aims have survived to the present (but with far more emphasis on the first, of course). The last of the four, very much the child of the kind of analyses undertaken in the three inner area studies, has since fallen by the wayside. No one now speaks of striking a balance between the inner cities on the one hand and outer cities and city regions on the other. It was never seriously tried (indeed, it was never seriously thought about) and certainly did not find favour with the incoming Conservative government in 1979. Any attempt to achieve such a balance after all would have required strong development controls as well as subsidised development opportunities. And whilst the latter were entirely consistent with government thinking, the former smacked of negative interventionism. (Only purists will quibble at the inconsistency here.)

By 1981 the purpose of the Urban Programme (by now incorporating Partnership and Programme Authority arrangements and the traditional Urban Programme) had come to be more succinctly stated as 'to assist in the regeneration of the most deprived urban areas, and covers industrial, environmental and recreational provision as well as specifically social projects' (Department of the Environment 1981a). We may safely assume that the 'assist in' was to avoid presenting too many hostages to fortune and to provide the same sort of plausibility insurance as the idea of 'bending'. More to the point however, there is no indication here of how these various projects will effect regeneration, or of what regeneration means – particularly in respect of inner city residents. It is not, after all, entirely facetious to ask what a regenerated inner city resident would look like. (Indeed, it is a mark of how far 'people' have been absent from recent inner city policy that we have to remind ourselves that they are what it is all about, unless the explosion of post-modernist office blocks on waterfronts all over the country is just the product of enterprise exhilaration.)

Even within the Urban Programme – that is, after the emergence of more specifically economic policies – the economic regeneration strategy came increasingly to the forefront. What had been said only coyly in 1981 was being stated more explicitly three years later. Schemes under the Urban Programme were to have three main aims:

> Securing economic regeneration, improving the physical environment and ensuring that local services and amenities are geared to the particular social needs of the local communities. *Priority should be given to projects aimed at economic regeneration.*
>
> (Department of the Environment 1984, emphasis added)

The mechanisms by which economic regeneration would reach into more general deprivation remained obscure – indeed, opaque might be a more appropriate word – but the next restatement of the aims of Urban Programme projects three years later at least gave a more explicit ideological twist to these aims and at the same time provided a glimpse of what the regenerated inner city resident should be like. Urban Programme projects therefore should:

- encourage *individual enterprise* and help local businesses, e.g. through providing managed workshops;
- improve the environment by improving derelict buildings and landscaping sites;
- encourage *self-help* and *reduce dependency on social services*, e.g. encouraging dual-use of schools and colleges for use by the community.

> (Department of the Environment 1987, para 4, emphases added)

Clearly this formulation of the aims of the Urban Programme has a very different flavour from that which preceded it by three years. Gone is any mention of meeting social needs. Instead the programme was to be about encouraging enterprise, promoting self-help and reducing welfare dependency. And so we have, for the first time, a clear indication of the enterprise culture beginning to steer the aims of the programme which at the same time appeared to be losing its needs-meeting focus.

By 1987, however, the Urban Programme had ceased to be at the forefront of inner city policy, and other programmes even more dedicated to the promotion of enterprise were being presented as the vanguard of policy. The same document that gave the enterprise flavour to the Urban Programme also outlined the government's objectives for urban policy in general, by which it meant 'bent' main programmes and rate support grant and also the aims of all DoE programmes collectively. The purpose of urban policy in general was:

- to improve employment prospects in the inner cities by increasing both job opportunities and the ability of those who live there to compete for them;
- to reduce the number of derelict sites and vacant buildings;
- to strengthen the social fabric of the inner city and encourage self-help;
- to reduce the number of people in acute housing stress.

(Department of the Environment 1987, para 1)

And of DoE initiatives, the same paper noted that their purpose was to:

- target assistance on the areas of greatest need, where results can be seen, and a stimulus given to wider regeneration;
- keep regulation and intervention by central and local government to a minimum, and concentrate activity on creating the right climate for investment and enterprise;
- build up business confidence by tackling dereliction, by pump priming investment, and by improving local labour skills;
- help make urban areas places where people want to live and industry wants to invest.

(Department of the Environment 1987, para 2)

Most (but not all) of the elements contained in subsequent statements of the aims of inner city policy in general were recorded in this catalogue. Certainly the flavour of policies was made quite explicit. Notwithstanding the reference to improving housing conditions, general urban policy and DoE programmes in particular were now about enterprise, economic regeneration, environmental improvement (to make the areas more attractive to inward *investment*), the promotion of self-help and strengthening the 'social fabric' which, given its juxtaposition with 'self-help', presumably means making people more independent, self-reliant, entrepreneurial and enterprising. (But then it could mean anything, or, more precisely, nothing.)

These statements of aims deserve further comment for reasons that have to do specifically with our own purpose here. Firstly, there can be no reading of these aims – of the Urban Programme in particular, of DoE programmes collectively, or of *urban policy in general* – that permits the government now to say that the aims of all inner city policy are *not* primarily about the promotion of enterprise and the stimulation of economic regeneration. Policies change of course, but as of 1992 nothing has been said to suggest that the government has changed its mind about what inner city policies are supposed to do. And however much the 'bending' card is played, the real message is clear from the hand that the government itself has dealt.

Secondly, and perhaps more subjectively, whilst reading these policy aims, it is necessary to remind oneself that they really are policy statements. There is (a strange phrase to use about a policy statement) something self-consciously arrogant about them. We have come, for good reason, to expect policy statements to be relatively dispassionate and dry and not to wear their ideological colours so openly on their sleeve. It is hard to avoid the conclusion that these statements of aims have more to do with pro-pounding a political doctrine than with recording a set of plausible and achievable goals – of whatever ideological slant. None of which makes the task of the policy analyst any easier. How is anyone going to be able to say to what extent these policies are working when the benchmark they have to work to is ideological fluff?

Some additional elements have been written into subsequent statements of the aims of inner city policy but, as we have noted, the flavour has remained largely unchanged. Both the *Action for Cities* and *People in Cities* brochures published in 1988 and 1990 respectively list policy purposes as being to:

- encourage enterprise and new businesses, and help existing businesses to grow stronger;
- improve people's job prospects, their motivation and skills;
- make areas attractive to residents and to business by
  - tackling dereliction
  - bringing buildings into use
  - preparing sites and encouraging development
  - improving the quality of housing;
- make inner city areas safe and attractive places to live and work.
  (Cabinet Office 1988: 5; Department of the Environment 1990b: 2)

This was the mixture much as before but with the addition of the 'safety' component which was specified more exactly in yet another brochure in the same year, as 'reducing crime' (see Department of the Environment 1989b; National Audit Office 1990: 7), and of another ingredient of 'enterprise man' – motivation.

Some of the aims outlined in the above and preceding lists are un-exceptionable; others, as we have noted, bear little resemblance to what we have come to expect of policy statements and among the more bizarre of the latter are those concerning inner city residents themselves. These docu-ments betray either a very patronising or a very dim view of the people who live in or near to areas which the government has designated as inner cities. They are people who need to learn more self-help, who are overly dependent on welfare, who constitute a weak social fabric and who are wanting in motivation. It is hard to escape the conclusion that so far as the government is concerned, the inner city problem consists in some measure of people who are inadequate – the antithesis in fact of 'enterprise man', thrusting, driven, effective, self-sufficient, self-improving, and – yes – *in re* that election victory oration – Conservative-voting.

What the foregoing review of ten years of policy statements demonstrates beyond doubt is that the idea of private-sector-led economic regeneration took root early in the 1980s and grew stronger through the decade, to the extent that it became (and remains) *the* inner city strategy. Emollient references to 'bending' notwithstanding, if we remove the economic regeneration strategy, the government does not have an inner city policy. Small, isolated items there may be that are not enterprise-focused, but they do not add up to a policy and they are dwarfed by the components of the main strategy. In evaluating enterprise and the promotion of the enterprise ethos therefore, we are evaluating the government's policy for the inner cities and for dealing with urban deprivation.

THE DoE AND THE INNER CITY PROBLEM

Descriptions of the inner city problem (the problem that the engine of enterprise is to solve or at least alleviate) are notably absent from recent departmental brochures in any other than the most general terms. As we have noted, poverty and deprivation, the chronically poor and the chronically ill and high dependency ratios do not get a mention. We must go back to a DoE publication of 1984 to find a more detailed specification – and even then it is a paraphrase of one published originally in the White Paper of 1977:

> the inner urban problem. . .was generally taken [by the White Paper] to be some combination of: decayed infrastructure; bad physical conditions; high levels of unemployment; limited job opportunities; and a concentration of people with social difficulties. Deprived urban areas also tend to include in their population a high proportion of ethnic minorities.
>
> (Department of the Environment 1984: 1)

Though better than much of what came later, this specification remains inadequate in a number of respects both for policy formulation and evaluation purposes. Its most serious deficiency as a problem specification around which practical policy could be formulated is the lack of any itemisation of the 'social difficulties' which inner city residents are alleged to have. We might fairly ask, 'what possible sort of policy could we put together to remove "social difficulties"?' An obvious candidate that springs to mind is the employment of more social workers (or 'agony aunts'?). But it is doubtful that this is what the drafters of the White Paper had in mind. Clearly, if there is a concentration of people with 'social difficulties', these need to be itemised. A second shortcoming is consequent upon the first. Without an itemisation of what 'social difficulties' includes, it is impossible to establish why such concentrations exist and what has caused them (if anything). There is no indication for example of whether a causal link is supposed between decayed infrastructure, bad physical conditions, high levels of unemployment and poor job opportunities on the one hand and 'social difficulties' on the other. Might it be (we are hypothesising what might have been in the minds of the drafters) that the spatial coexistence of social difficulties and other factors is simply coincidental, that the people with them would have them wherever they lived? This is important for two reasons: firstly as a formulation in policy makers' minds that influenced (or not) the policy output; and secondly as a specification of what really is the case which will be crucial for evaluating the effectiveness of policy. The third deficiency relates to the question of spatial concentration. Only in respect of people with social difficulties is the notion of 'concentration' used. We are left to surmise therefore that it is the relative concentration of the other factors also which characterises inner cities. But this creates difficulties. The problem specification that we have *implies* that inner cities are specifiable independently of the spatial concentration of the factors listed, in so far as they are thought to have 'some combination of them'. We are not told however what this independent specification is. But then if conversely inner cities are to be identified as those areas with relative concentrations of these factors (not all of which will be near to city centres) we have the difficulty that not all, and perhaps not most, of these factors will show the same spatial concentrations. There are a variety of solutions to this problem, most of which would use some notion of the 'best fit' of separate but overlapping concentrations, but the problem specification as it stands is devoid not only of a solution but of any indication even of an awareness of the difficulties.

URBAN DEPRIVATION ITEMISED

One of our main concerns is with the 'reach' of private-sector-led economic regeneration. We shall have something to say subsequently about whether the strategy of attracting investment is likely to achieve this specific end and about a diagnosis that rests heavily on the collapse of economic infrastructure, but more immediately we need a more comprehensive item-isation of urban deprivation than is provided in government department documents, and in particular the one we have examined above.

Briefly to restate our purpose: we want to establish whether and to what extent the enterprise solution to the inner city problem – the use of levered private sector investment to effect economic regeneration – will reduce urban deprivation, by which we mean in general terms that body of dis-welfares from which some people who register varying degrees of spatial concentration, appear to suffer. We do this for two reasons: firstly because notwithstanding the silence on the matter of recent government brochures, urban deprivation *is* an important component of the inner city problem; and secondly because we are making the not unreasonable assumption that economic regeneration is not being promoted just for its own sake but also because of a belief that it will have an impact on the diswelfares of inner city residents. We cannot therefore achieve our purpose without firstly detailing what constitutes urban deprivation.

The following characteristics are all associated in some way with the 'inner city problem', either individually or in a variety of combinations.

a) Characteristics associated with people or households:
  – poverty and income support dependency
  – unemployment
  – chronic unemployment (long-term or frequent)
  – the unskilled and the under-skilled
  – one-parent families
  – large families or households
  – the elderly (and especially the lone elderly)
  – the sick and the chronically sick
  – families in need of social work support.
b) Environmental factors:
  – poor physical environment and physical dilapidation
  – environmental pollution
  – crime and fear of crime
  – social tension.
c) Housing factors:
  – poor quality housing and physically dilapidated housing
  – overcrowded housing
  – housing with only shared amenities.
d) Educational factors:
  – physically run-down schools
  – poor teaching
  – low levels of educational attainment.
e) Service provision:
  – poor or inadequate health services
  – poor environmental services
  – poor financial services (hire purchase, loans, mortgages).

f) Economic and financial factors:
   – decayed economic infrastructure
   – poor and inadequate tax base
   – a high dependency ratio.

The list may not be entirely comprehensive but it probably includes the great majority and certainly the most important components of deprivation. Neither would there be unanimity on all the items on the list or on the omissions. (There is nothing here about the social fabric or want of motivation.) But we believe that there is enough in the list for most people with an interest in the inner cities to recognise much that is familiar.

As a description of urban deprivation or the inner city problem, the list is too stark. For it to serve our purposes, it requires some elaboration. The categorisation of items is largely self-explanatory: there are factors which attach to individuals, families or households which may in themselves be disadvantaging or which are likely to provoke a greater risk of disadvantage; there are characteristics of some inner city areas themselves which constitute diswelfares or depress the quality of life; there are welfare consumption goods such as housing and education which affect both quality of life and future prospects; there is a range of other services, the poor quality of which may depress quality of life; and finally there are economic and financial factors which will include the damaged economic infrastructure which, as we have seen, is argued to be the root cause of the inner city problem, and, partly consequent upon this, an inadequate local tax base upon which to support relatively high welfare spending.

The first of these categories – what we have called 'characteristics associated with people or households' – deserves some further elucidation. Not all the items here are taxonomically identical and they would not all, for this reason, find the same place in the logic of the impact of policy. Some, such as poverty, unemployment, sickness and families in need of social work support, are, in varying degrees, 'problematic' in themselves. Others, such as low-skill, one-parent and large families and the elderly, are not inherently problematic but appear on the list for two reasons. Firstly, individuals or households with these characteristics are at greater risk of suffering diswelfares such as poverty, unemployment, illness and insecurity (see for example Holman 1970; Rutter and Madge 1976; Holman 1978; Coffield *et al.* 1980; MacGregor 1981, Chapter 3), and secondly, there are relative concentrations of such potentially vulnerable groups in some inner city areas.[1] Whilst it is logical therefore to assert that policy (of whatever kind) ought to be concerned with reducing poverty, unemployment, and the problems of 'at risk' families, the same cannot be said in respect of large or one-parent families or the elderly. The list therefore is only what it purports to be – an itemisation of characteristics associated with what is commonly called the 'inner city problem'. It contains a number of interrelated items to which any policy, if it is to be successful, must be sensitive.

Our itemisation of urban deprivation is therefore not grounded in any set of assumptions about the nature of the causal relationships between interdependent items (other than to justify the inclusion of some items on the basis of their indicating higher levels of risk) and neither is it dependent on any particular idea or theory about the causes of inner city deprivation. Whatever the causes, these are some of the manifestations. The items in Section a) of the list therefore on p. 51 (and indeed, all other sections) would still be there whether we subscribed to a 'filter-down' and 'residualisation' thesis about the inner city (see for example Harvey 1973, Chapter 2; Johnston 1980, Chapter 6; Knox 1982, Chapter 3) or one that favoured a 'cycle of deprivation' and 'culture of poverty' explanation (see Wedge and Prosser 1973; Coffield *et al.* 1980; Essen and Wedge 1982) or the economic infrastructure approach.

There remains one aspect of the itemisation of 'urban deprivation' that requires further comment here. We have variously referred to the list as being made up of components of 'urban deprivation' and of items that characterise the 'inner city problem'. Elsewhere we have referred to 'urban deprivation' as one component of the inner city problem. It remains to clarify this apparent anomaly. We have characterised urban deprivation as a body of diswelfares that affect people who live in varying degrees of spatial concentration. (Many of the same diswelfares occur outside cities and are spatially dissipated, but it is their relative concentration in some areas that gives rise to the particular policy responses we are dealing with.) Given this formulation, some items on the list (decayed economic infrastructure, inadequate local tax base) may appear more like causes than effects and not to constitute diswelfares in the same way that poverty, unemployment, bad housing and inadequate services do. To that extent, they would constitute part of the inner city problem but not of urban deprivation. Whether the economic infrastructure and the tax base constitute causes of deprivation or are themselves part of the diswelfares that inner city residents face is largely a semantic matter however, and we shall maintain the distinction between items under f) (p. 52) and all others on the list, only in so far as argument requires it.

We shall not elaborate further on the individual components of deprivation: it is not our purpose to dilate on the meaning of poverty and how it can be measured, or on what constitutes poor schooling or underachievement or the need for social work support. The subsequent evaluation of the strategy of economic regeneration will require that some of the components of deprivation will need to be elucidated but for present purposes, the above itemisation serves to demonstrate the nature and variability of the phenomena that the enterprise strategy must have some impact on if it is to be deemed to be successful. And again, lest it be argued that we are making too many and too extravagant demands on the enterprise strategy, it has to be emphasised that so far as the spatial concentration of combinations of components of deprivation (i.e. the inner city dimension) is concerned, if we exclude the economic regeneration programmes of current inner city policy, there is very little left either of that policy or of mainstream policies that is directed particularly at urban deprivation.

Few, if any, of the characteristics we have identified as components of urban deprivation are peculiar to those areas that we call 'inner cities'. What we call the 'inner city dimension' above derives from the relative spatial concentrations of varying combinations of these components in some areas which are often, but by no means always, located near to the central business districts of medium and large-sized cities. It is the relative concentration of combinations of deprivations that characterises the 'inner city problem', rather than anything peculiarly different about the deprivations themselves. Though this may appear to be stating the obvious, it is not always clear that those responsible for making policy have grasped the fact. If it is only the *concentration* of mixes of otherwise common and widely found deprivations that occasions a policy response that is unique to those areas of concentration (and does not apply to the same deprivations when found elsewhere), then this is clearly imbuing spatial concentration with a great deal of particular significance. And when we add to this the fact that the particular mix of deprivations may vary considerably from one city to another, it appears that even *more* weight is being attached to concentration itself. We shall return to this topic when we consider spatial concentration and the idea of an inner city economy. Our next task however is to catalogue current (and immediate past) inner city programmes and policies and their intended purposes so that we can identify how much and which parts of the whole are designed to promote the economic regeneration strategy. We shall then be in a position to specify more precisely what ends this strategy is intended to achieve and to hypothesise on the mechanisms by which it might achieve them.

INNER CITY PROGRAMMES AND INITIATIVES

Inner city programmes and programmes that have relevance to, or are partially targeted at, the inner cities, have blossomed and wilted with remarkable frequency over the past five years. Any attempt to catalogue them therefore will soon be out of date. There has also been a tendency, particularly since the *Action for Cities* umbrella was unfurled in 1988, for a very wide range of policies with seemingly little to do with the inner cities (such as the National Curriculum for schools) to be brought within its shelter. Drawing up a reasonably accurate, comprehensive, but realistic list of inner-city-related schemes therefore is not as easy a task as might appear. The components of inner city policy are fairly fluid. The following list of inner-city-related schemes, broken down by the responsible government department, is confined to programmes that are inner-city specific or which have an identifiable inner city component. It excludes other programmes that have been mentioned in government brochures and which may have some incidental effect in inner city areas but which have no specific inner area component.

Department of the Environment [2]

Urban development corporations
Urban Programme
City action teams
Enterprise zones (only one designation after December 1987)
Simplified planning zones
City Grant
Land registers
Derelict Land Grant
Priority Estates Project
Estate Action
Housing action trusts
Garden festivals
Housing investment programmes (inner city component from 1990/91)

Department of Employment

Enterprise Allowance Scheme
Small Firms Service
Managed workshops
Loan guarantee schemes
Youth Training Scheme
Job clubs
Employment Training Programme
Restart Programme
Action for Jobs
Schools/Industry Compact

Department of Trade and Industry

Task forces
Local enterprise agencies
Regional enterprise grants
Regional Selective Assistance

Home Office

Section 11 grants
Safer cities

Department of Education and Science

Pickup Programme
City Technology Colleges

Cabinet

'Ministerial Adoption' (nine cities)

(Department of the Environment, Department of Trade and Industry and Department of Employment 1987; Department of the Environment and Department of Employment 1987; Department of the Environment 1987; Cabinet Office 1988; Department of the Environment 1988a; Department of the Environment 1989b; Department of the Environment 1990a and b.)

The constituent purposes of all these items fall into four broad categories:

– investment and business promotion;
– employment training and education;
– land reclamation and environmental improvement;
– housing improvement.

Two schemes – the Safer Cities Project and Section 11 grants – do not fall easily into any of these categories but the safer cities initiative, designed to reduce crime, and the fear of crime could be seen in part at least as an aspect of (perceived) environmental improvement. There is only an approximate association between these categories and the departments responsible for sponsoring each item.

There is no clear distinction among these categories between those that are essentially concerned with promoting private sector investment (and hence 'enterprise') and those with different purposes. The first category –

investment and business promotion – is clearly about nurturing enterprise in the inner cities, and housing improvement equally clearly is not primarily so concerned. The other two categories are not so easily placed, but in the main it can be said that land reclamation and environmental improvements are largely to do with facilitating private investment (although not always in the inner cities). How best to treat employment training and education for our purposes is less clear. Two alternatives present themselves. The first is that high levels of unemployment in the inner cities (because of lack of skills) is an unnecessary evil in itself (or it causes riots) and must for that reason alone be dealt with. The second is that private-sector regeneration depends upon the availability of a larger pool of trained workers without which its growth would be frustrated. In this case, the former would depend upon the latter and the various training schemes would be undertaken to enable private-sector investment to go forward. The concomitant of this, of course, is that if a sufficiently large pool of trained workers already existed (that could, for example, be imported into the inner cities), then there would be no need for training programmes. Unfortunately, what looks at first sight like an empirical question contains strong ideological undertones. In practice, concern from a number of quarters has centred around the danger that inner city residents will not benefit from the employment growth that follows new investment either because incoming firms will bring their own work-force with them (if they are relocating) or they will attract already skilled and trained labour from outside the inner cities (see, for example, House of Commons Employment Committee 1988a; Docklands Consultative Committee 1988; Whyatt 1988). And for inner city residents themselves, it probably matters little whether the skills training on offer is primarily to service private sector investment or for other reasons of justice or utility; it may still provide the means to a better quality of life and some greater security. If, therefore, the private sector regeneration strategy is to work to the benefit of inner city residents, it must be allied to education and training programmes that will provide those in the labour force with the necessary skills. Given that there is no *overall* skills shortage among firms that might relocate or develop in inner city areas, however, it would appear that training and education are not a *necessary* component of inner city economic regeneration at present.

We can now classify the various inner-city-related schemes according to their main purposes.

Investment and business promotion

Urban Development Corporations
Urban Programme (also contains social and environmental components)

City Action Teams
Enterprise Zones
Enterprise Allowance Scheme
Small Firms Service
Managed Workshops
Loan Guarantee Scheme
Task forces
Local enterprise agencies
Regional enterprise grants
Regional Selective Assistance

Land reclamation and environmental improvement

City Grant
Simplified Planning Zones
Land Registers
Derelict Land Grant
Garden Festivals
(Safer Cities)

Employment training and education

Employment Training Programme
Restart Programme
Action For Jobs
Schools/Industry Compact
Job Clubs
Youth Training Scheme
Pickup Programme
City Technology Colleges

Housing improvement

Priority Estates Project
Estate Action
Housing Action Trusts
Housing Investment Programme

Other

Section 11 grants
'Ministerial Adoption'

With the possible exception of derelict land grants, all the schemes in the first two categories are aimed solely or primarily at promoting private sector economic regeneration; that is, seventeen of the thirty-two schemes listed. A further eight schemes – those concerned with training and education – are indirectly concerned with enterprise promotion, leaving only the four housing schemes and the two 'miscellaneous' not connected with the 'enterprise' solution in some way (though it should be noted that the Urban Programme does contain a 'social' element as well as 'economic' and 'environmental' elements).

In terms of the overall proportion of inner city schemes therefore, it is clear that the government is putting its weight unequivocally behind private sector regeneration – just as its publicity and policy promotion would have us believe. Further than this, as we have noted, the Urban development corporations – an example *par excellence* of the enterprise strategy (see Cabinet Office 1988: 12; Department of the Environment 1990a: 4) – have been, and still are, being promoted as the most important and at the forefront of all inner city strategies. However, none of this tells us where the bulk of inner city funds are being spent.[3] The schemes we have listed vary a great deal in size and the resources allocated to them. Some, like the City Action Teams and the task forces, have very small expenditure consequences; others, like the Urban Development Corporations, are large and growing (at least, until 1991/92). Unfortunately, because so many of these schemes are not confined exclusively to the inner cities (only an unspecified amount of their total allocation being targeted there), it is not possible to calculate with any accuracy the relative proportions of total inner city funds that may be apportioned to each of the four function heads we have identified. The following data are therefore only illustrative but serve to add emphasis to the picture painted above of the dominance of the enterprise strategy within inner city policy as a whole.

Estimated expenditure for the three main participating departments on inner city schemes in 1988/89 were as follows:

Department of the Environment : £1,130m
Department of Employment Group : £1,120m
Department of Trade and Industry : £220m

(National Audit Office 1990: 7. No figure is given for the Home Office. Figures for the Department of Transport and the Scottish and Welsh Offices are not included here.)

All of the Trade and Industry expenditure may be counted as enterprise-related, as the lists above indicate. Secondly, virtually all of the employment expenditure may also be allotted to the training and education head (along with an unspecifiable amount from education). The environment figure includes amounts for housing and the 'social' component of the Urban Programme (and for the 'environment' component, but this, like other DoE 'environment' schemes, we can count as *primarily* concerned with economic regeneration). It is not possible to specify a value for housing expenditure in the inner cities (the government expenditure plans and the National Audit Office Report both being silent on this) but a rough approximation for the social and housing components of the Urban Programme is possible. Provision by the Department of the Environment in 1988/89 for the Urban Programme was £183m, to which must be added further provision of £101m by the Departments of Education and Science, Health and Transport. In that year, 24 per cent of this total Urban Programme provision went on social projects and a further 9 per cent to housing projects, giving £95m for these broadly non-enterprise projects and £189m for economic and environmental projects. If we then make the (heroic) assumption that the apportionment of Urban Programme funds under the three heads was similar for the DoE as for all departmentally combined programme funds, then some 33 per cent of Environment's £183m went on social and housing projects and the remainder (£121m) on enterprise-related projects. Of the total DoE inner cities expenditure of £1,130m, therefore, only something like £61m is likely to have gone on non-enterprise-related activities in the inner cities.

Taken together, therefore, these figures demonstrate a very marked bias in inner city expenditure patterns towards enterprise-related schemes, and this remains the case even if we exclude education and training which, as we have already noted, may or may not be considered a necessary concomitant of the enterprise strategy. It is not just presentationally therefore that private sector-led economic regeneration constitutes the foremost component of inner city policy; the great majority of all the schemes that make up that policy, and the lion's share of the resources devoted to it, are directed at the same strategy.

We have now completed our initial tasks of itemising urban deprivation and of identifying the nature and extent of policy practices ranged against it. The former has been shown to be multivariate and characterised by conditions affecting people, households and families, conditions that may predispose to dependency and insecurity, environmental factors, the quality of services, housing conditions and economic fragility. It is a daunting catalogue and it makes the manner of the recent presentation of policy look not only complacent but even contemptuous. Against this hydra is pitted a large number of individual schemes, the majority of which have a single narrow strategic focus – the economic regeneration of the areas in which the many components of urban deprivation show relative spatial concentration. Clearly, the reach and scope of the enterprise strategy is expected to be very wide. In short, it is expected to achieve many things on many fronts. The next task must therefore be to articulate by what means such a single-minded strategy can accomplish so much. Or failing that, how its proponents think it can.

NOTES

1   The question of the relative concentration of some or all of these characteristics in some inner city areas and whether inner city areas can usefully be defined independently of such concentrations is a much broader one that we shall pursue later in this and in Chapter 4.
2   A number of the initiatives carried by the DoE will in future be transferred to the new Urban Regeneration Agency announced in the Queen's Speech on 6 May 1992 and first mooted in the Conservative Party manifesto earlier in the year (Conservative Party 1992). Its main task will be to attract developers to derelict or unused sites (though not necessarily in the inner cities). It will act in partnership with private sector developers but is empowered to act as a developer in its own right. It will also have powers of compulsory purchase. The legislation that will bring the Agency into being (the Housing, Land, and Urban Development Bill) has, at the time of writing, yet to reach its second reading.
3   Even calculating total inner city expenditure can be a hazardous task. Probably the best estimate would include the 'Urban Block' of expenditure for which the DoE is responsible (£789 million in 1990/91) supplemented by the 'inner city' elements of the budgets of the four other participating departments (DTI, DE, DES and Home Office), though even here, what constitutes an 'inner city element' can be a moveable feast.

4   The logic of the enterprise strategy

The immediate products of economic regeneration are plain enough; they adorn nearly every page of recent government brochures on inner city policy, the new marinas, office blocks, refurbished warehouses, landscaped derelict sites and so on. But they are (it is hoped) only the visible manifestations of the essence of recovery: a more buoyant local economy and, most important for our purposes, more new jobs. (Output measures for Urban Development Corporations used in government sources are more usually square metres of land reclaimed and of office and other development space created, the gearing ratio achieved and, on occasion, numbers of dwelling units completed. See for example Department of the Environment 1988a; 1989b; 1990a. Such sources tend to be more coy about the numbers of new jobs created, for reasons that we shall subsequently discuss.)

So far as the schemes we have identified as either for investment and business promotion or for land reclamation and environmental improvement are concerned therefore, the general purposes are similar. Land reclamation and environmental improvements are carried out primarily to provide more attractive areas in which investment can locate (which is not to say that there is *no* domestic environmental improvement or reclamation for housing purposes). Infrastructure works are normally provided as part of the public subsidy to attract business. Relaxed planning requirements serve the same function, and the variety of loan schemes and financial help for small firms are designed either to support existing businesses in the inner cities or to help local unemployed people to start up new businesses.

There is a common theme then to all these interrelated schemes, though it comes in varying degrees of sophistication (or opacity). At its simplest it is about increasing the volume of business activity and hence the number of jobs in a specified area or available to people who live in that area. A more sophisticated version talks about regenerating the economies of inner city areas (see for example Eversley 1980; Brownrigg 1983; Solesbury 1987;

Turok 1987). The former would be subsumed within the latter, but regenerating inner city economies is presumably intended to convey more than just increasing investment activity and the numbers of jobs. How much more is intended by the revival of inner city economies and how much more this means in practice, we shall examine later in this chapter. For the moment, we shall pursue the easier logic involved in business and job creation without entering the more turbulent waters of inner city economies. Apart from some domestic environmental improvements and housing provision then, the collective aims of all the schemes we have identified as being in pursuit of 'enterprise' are quite limited. Yet from these limited aims (business and job creation) extensive benefits are expected to flow: the alleviation (at least) of a wide and heterogeneous range of deprivations and dependencies. How will this happen?

The precise mechanisms by which economic regeneration will reduce (no one has claimed elimination) urban deprivation as constituted by the large number and wide variety of characteristics we have identified, have never been articulated either by government departments responsible for implementing the policies of regeneration nor by commentators on the inner cities. No doubt civil servants in the relevant departments would want to enter a disclaimer at this point. We will do it for them: government policy statements have never claimed that the 'enterprise solution' will solve (reduce) all the ills we have identified as urban deprivation; we have 'set them up'. This is true only literally however, in so far as departments responsible for policy have shied away from specifying what their policies are intended to achieve; they are responsible for providing their own hostages to fortune. What we have identified as 'urban deprivation' is that range of problems found in varying combinations in inner city areas. It is reasonable to assume that they are problems that inner city policies ought to address. There is little, either in terms of numbers of schemes or of resources, that is not directed at the enterprise strategy. If therefore this strategy is not directed at urban deprivation, there is little that is. Either current policy is not in the main concerned with urban deprivation or it is – and through the enterprise strategy. We more generously assume the latter.

There will be some immediate spin-off for inner city residents from economic regeneration. They will come largely in the form of environmental improvements to their surroundings. Most of the environmental improvements brought about by schemes under that heading will not however be on a domestic or community scale and will not immediately affect the environment at the neighbourhood level. The bulk of these resources has gone and will continue to go on large-scale land reclamation and preparation for commercial, office, and light industrial use. The more grandiose schemes in the London and Merseyside docklands and in

Trafford Park for example have all been in preparation for inward investment, not for providing a better domestic environment (see London Docklands Development Corporation 1990a; Trafford Park Development Corporation 1990a; Merseyside Development Corporation 1990). That being said, *some* domestic environmental improvements will accrue from the enterprise strategy. Far and away the most important product of the strategy however, so far as impact on deprivation is concerned, would be the creation of new jobs and it is on this that we shall concentrate. The decisive question therefore will be how far the creation of new jobs will reach into and have an impact on the multifarious nature of urban deprivation. The answer has to be speculative, there being little but hunches, conventional wisdom and not a little wishful thinking to draw on. (There is a *sine qua non* to all this of course, and that is that the strategy *would* create new jobs and that these jobs would go to the previously unemployed inner city labour force – however that might be defined.)

We wish to be as specific as speculation will allow in detailing the potential reach of new job creation, and for this purpose we shall count in the itemised constituents of deprivation as they might or might not be touched by ripple effects. By definition, its immediate impact will be on unemployment levels[1] and this will serve to reduce (or eliminate) poverty in those households with a member in the labour force previously unemployed. Those suffering from chronic unemployment and (an overlap category) those with few or no skills, will not however necessarily benefit from job creation unless a significant proportion of the jobs are unskilled (and often low paid) or a sufficient and suitable volume of training is implemented to equip the local labour force to take the jobs. This, as we have seen, is an important component of the overall inner city strategy; without it (and its being successful), the enterprise strategy will not reach the majority in the labour force who are most at risk of frequent or long-term unemployment. Other at-risk groups in the compass of deprivation – one-parent and large families – would benefit in the same way if a previously unemployed member gained employment, but they might remain at relatively greater risk of poverty or insecurity. The elderly and the sick would benefit from trickle effects if a household member upon whom they were dependent or partially dependent were to get a job, but this in itself would do little for other dimensions of their deprivation such as poor or inadequate services or an environment that was perceived as hostile. Similarly, additional income from employment might alleviate some of the difficulties which bring families into contact with social services departments, but only rarely is it likely to be the case that this would provide an adequate resolution to all their difficulties.

The various characteristics of deprivation associated with people or households do not always, or even usually, occur in isolation. Not only are they sometimes ecologically related (in the sense of occurring in relatively high frequency in the same areas),[2] they also occur in combination within the same households and families (see for example Holman 1978, Chapter 1; Brown and Madge 1982, Part II).[3] The same is true of many of the components of deprivation that fall under other headings in our itemised list. To attempt to identify all possible types of interaction and their potential mutually reinforcing effects would be an impossible task, and all that it is possible to say here is that alleviation of some components (as a result of gaining employment for example) may also reduce general pressure, dependency, or insecurity resulting from multiple effects at the household level. Thus reduction in deprivation at the personal or household level *may* have knock-on effects on other manifestations of deprivation under other heads. A decaying environment, stressful housing conditions or poor services may be made more bearable by the relief of anxiety over unemployment or lack of money even though they remain unaltered themselves by job creation. Any more direct effects of the investment strategy are likely to be more muted however.

The second category of deprivation components that we identified were 'environmental factors', and we need not dwell long on these improvements because we have already noted that the bulk of land reclamation and improvement will be in preparation for investment. It may therefore facilitate job creation and indirectly alleviate deprivation in the ways outlined above, but it will not effect any direct change. There will, in addition, be some domestic environmental improvements and to the extent that these improvements render neighbourhood environments more pleasant, they will more directly reduce some of the manifestations of deprivation under the environment head. Nothing under this head however is likely seriously to reduce levels of crime or – probably more important – the fear of crime. The same may be said of 'social tension' – a source of excitement for some and dread for others – particularly the elderly. As a component of urban deprivation it is probably of little significance, if only because it is confined (probably) to a small number of areas and its intensity is spasmodic.[4] Where there really is social tension (which in reality is usually a euphemism for racial tension) it can of course be an extremely debilitating environmental cost to bear for those for whom it is not a source of anger and excitement. The solutions to the problems of crime levels (and fear of them) and of racial tension (if there are any available) must be found elsewhere, even though they constitute part of the environmental costs of inner cities.

There are, as we have noted, housing components to the overall inner cities policy package, but they sit apart from the investment strategy. This strategy itself will not, and is not, designed to have a direct influence on housing and housing conditions in the inner cities however, and as such we must assume that housing components of deprivation fall largely outside its reach.

Nor is it likely that the enterprise strategy will in any direct way improve the physical fabric of inner city schools, the poor levels of teaching found in some of them, or the relatively low levels of educational achievement of many pupils who attend them. Outside the area of training, on which a significant portion of inner city resources are expended, there is little besides the schools/industry compacts – themselves very small in scale – in the enterprise strategy that will reach into educational deprivation.

The penultimate category of components of deprivation that we have listed relates to service provision and, in particular, poor or inadequate health and environmental services (a common but by no means universal characteristic of inner cities) and, often as a result of reputational effects, poor financial services of one sort or another. Proponents of the enterprise strategy will argue that the last of these is just the sort of adverse reputational effect that a decayed economic infrastructure will create and that it can be 'turned around' as the enterprise strategy begins to bite. Indeed, is this not just what the enterprise strategy is all about: breathing new economic confidence into areas in which its stock has all but disappeared? In fact, the – at first – unpromising idea of financial services and credit confidence may prove to be an important diagnostic of the success of the investment strategy. The idea of financial confidence in an area (on the part of, for example, lending institutions) is a somewhat amorphous one to grasp. More readily envisaged is the ability of individuals and households to obtain credit of one form or another. What the former requires us to accept is that the latter – the same people in the same situations – will find it easier to obtain credit *because* the stock of confidence in the economic health of the area has risen as a result of regeneration. But is not credit-worthiness a possession of individuals rather than areas? And if the personal position of inner city residents has not been changed by economic regeneration, will they find credit easier to obtain just because financial confidence in the *area* is more buoyant? Within the total scope of urban deprivation the difficulties of obtaining credit may be of relatively small significance, but it does raise in a microcosm the logical uncertainties about how even successful economic regeneration may alleviate deprivation where its manifestation is most painful – at the individual and household levels.

Of other inadequacies of service provision – in health and environmental – and possibly other public services – little need be said; there seems little reason to believe that a private sector investment strategy will have any perceptible impact on these. Our sixth and final category of deprivations is of a different kind to the others. We have already noted the ambiguity about whether economic and financial factors are best treated as deprivations from which inner city residents suffer or as the causes of at least some of the other deprivations. Three components have been identified under this heading. The first is indeed the primary purpose of this strategy – to revitalise a decayed economic infrastructure. The other two require more comment. The high dependency ratio which, as calculated for any given area, is the collective result of a relative concentration of the personal and family deprivations or insecurities already considered, would be improved (that is, the ratio would be reduced) by a decrease in unemployment in the area. Its reduction is therefore dependent upon an increase in the jobs available to inner city residents and their ability to take them up, which in turn would require the provision and take-up of relevant training pro-grammes. The third component, the tax base of a given area, creates problems of its own for our analysis, if only because its determinants lie mainly outside inner city policy. It is not our intention to encroach on the realm of local government finance – there are others better qualified for this task.[5] Present purposes will be served by noting that before the introduction of the Uniform Business Rate in 1989, local authorities had a great deal more autonomy over their local tax revenues (and expenditures) and this gave real meaning to their industrial and commercial profile. Since 1989 and the imposition of a 'level playing field' however, this autonomy has been severely restricted and local authorities are no longer in a position to harvest any local tax gain from increased local investment. The mechanics of regeneration therefore no longer include the possibility of higher ex-penditure levels by local authorities to relieve deprivation, funded from a more robust tax base. Regeneration must now therefore do its job by employment creation and whatever impact it can make on the 'inner city economy'. This situation raises the more general question of the relative value and importance of local autonomy in expenditure to reduce deprivation and whether this should, or ought, to be a component of the enterprise strategy.

If the enterprise strategy is to be successful in reducing urban depri-vation therefore it will have to be by means of a reduction of dependency, insecurity and poverty as a result of the previously unemployed gaining employment from the new jobs created – the so called 'trickle down effect' (see Archbishop of Canterbury's Commission on Urban Priority Areas 1985: 205)[6] and by such indirect effects as may stem from bolstering inner city economies (of which more later). Assuming, for the purposes of argument, that the immediate aims of the enterprise strategy – the attraction of businesses to, and the creation of more jobs in inner city areas – are met, the logic of the trickle effect must still be qualified by the possibility that the 'new' jobs might not go to the previously unemployed in the inner city (because they do not have the necessary qualifications or because the jobs are imported complete with incumbent) and by the uncertainties of the *domestic* (re-) distribution of resources if jobs do go to inner city residents. Given that one of the distinguishing features of many inner city areas is their high dependency ratio and the relatively large numbers of people not in the work-force, we may be asking for too much of any trickle effect from employment gains.

THE IMPORTANCE OF A DISCRETE SPACE

Policy is ill served by the very ideas of 'inner cities' and 'inner city areas'. The first inner city policy, the Urban Programme, was founded on an (often unarticulated) notion of residual pockets of deprivation in spatial concentration (see Edwards and Batley 1978). The key components were deprivation as a social pathology and relatively discrete spatial pockets. We have escaped from the first of these assumptions as earlier chapters have shown, but the legacy of spatial concentration still informs – indeed to some extent underpins – present thinking. We shall reserve judgement on the potential policy implications of the signal importance that is attached to 'space' in the enterprise strategy to a later chapter; our concern here – as elsewhere in this chapter – is to draw out the logic of the strategy.

There are three dimensions to the area problem that are relevant so far as an evaluation of the effectiveness of enterprise is concerned. The first concerns the degree of spatial concentration of components of deprivation both singly and in combination. The second is about the idea of an 'inner city economy' and the extent of its spatial discreteness. And the third, and more directly policy related, is whether policies that rely on designating discrete areas can ever work if the premises underlying them on the first two dimensions turn out to be wrong.

The degree of spatial concentration of deprivation itself raises a number of related problems for policy. Firstly, there is the question of whether the spatial concentration of people suffering from any one – or more crucially – any combination of the components of deprivation we have identified is so great as to make the targeting of policies at these areas of concentration an effective and efficient means of tackling *most* deprivation. The obvious, though not particularly helpful, response, of course, is that it depends on how big the areas are, either for the purposes of identifying concentrations or of designation for policy attention. But if, in order to capture the majority of the deprived, the designated areas have to be very large, then not only is the precision of resource targeting very blunt but the designated areas are going to contain very large numbers of the non-deprived who will also be the beneficiaries of policy. This makes neither for efficiency nor effectiveness. The work of Holtermann as later developed by Townsend on the degree of concentration of people experiencing a number of deprivations (though now two decades old) clearly demonstrated by analysis at the enumeration district level, that this concentration was in fact very low (though variable) for all individual components of deprivation measured, and very low indeed for combinations of components (Holtermann 1975, 1978; Townsend 1976). On this analysis, even a generous definition of inner cities would exclude the great majority of the deprived and to capture even a half of deprived people by spatial targeting, we would have to designate nearly 50 per cent of the country's land area. Those small residual pockets of deprivation so attractive to the policy strategist turn out to be neither small nor residual.

What we are dealing with in inner city areas are *relative* concentrations of some components of urban deprivation. As a means of helping the *majority* of the deprived however, policies that rely on designating and concentrating resources in these areas (even generously defined), must fail. The rationale for inner city (as opposed to deprivation) policies however must be that they are *not* concerned with the majority of the deprived but rather with areas that not only have relative concentrations but also within which there are self-reinforcing spatial effects which mark them out as having particular and peculiar problems and distinguish them from other areas containing deprived people. And so we arrive at the notion that it is not the degree of spatial concentration of deprivations (singly or in combination) that makes inner cities discrete entities, but rather their own special internal dynamics (see Robson 1988: 43). Now the problem with this rationale is that it necessarily involves us in deriving causal associations from ecological data. The mere conjunction in one area of a number of 'deprivation factors' is no evidence in itself of any cumulative effect or causal interaction.

None the less it is tempting, and we are all guilty of it at one time or another. After all, is it not common sense that poverty, poor education, lack of jobs, low attainment and low expectations will interact and reinforce one another; that poor housing and a dismal environment will compound the sense of hopelessness and that financial institutions will not fall over themselves to lend or invest money in such areas when there are richer and more secure pickings a few miles down the road? The problem is, however, that apart from a few ethnographic studies there is little hard evidence as to the nature and extent of reinforcing spatial effects.

Much is made, in the language of enterprise-driven regeneration of the idea of the 'inner city economy', and it plays a key role in the logic of the enterprise strategy. Our evaluation in subsequent chapters will have to consider whether inner city economies are being regenerated but also, and more fundamentally, whether the concept itself will stand up to close scrutiny. Much of the logic of the enterprise strategy relies upon there being entities that can be called inner city economies which are capable of regeneration. Yet the concept itself remains undefined and unspecified and we shall need to flesh it out before we can trace the logic of regeneration that depends so heavily upon it.

The idea of an inner city economy suggests an economy that is relatively discrete and spatially confined to or functionally particular to the inner city. It suggests an economy that is relatively insulated from other economic activity (in the city, region, country and internationally) and which will provide livelihood and sustenance for the residents of the area. Furthermore (though this is a rather more tenuous assumption), its economic isolation implies that the economy itself will be sustained by the residents who will feed back into it resources that they extracted in the form of wages.

Now it has to be said that nowhere can be found such a description of an inner city economy. What we have provided here remains speculation, but the logic of economic regeneration requires that inner city economies conform to something like this specification. Given this sort of specification however, the nature of the inner city problem becomes more easily grasped and its remedy self-evident. If there are relatively insulated economies which supply the life-blood of inner cities, then it is clear that their demise or degeneration will be responsible for many of the problems that afflict these areas. And if the cause of the problems is so clearly focused then so may also be the solution: logic dictates that the inner city economies be regenerated.

Such a diagnosis is not incompatible with what is already known about the demise of the inner cities, but neither is it fully congruent. The main causes of decay are well known and documented as we have already noted – selective population loss, the exodus of companies (partly in response to decentralisation policies) and the death of others, traditionally low skill levels and hence high unemployment rates and so on (see for example Gripaios 1977; Dicken and Lloyd 1978; Cambridge Economic Policy Review 1982; Fothergill and Gudgin 1982; Healey and Clark 1983; Spence and Frost 1983; Buck *et al.* 1986; Lever and Moore 1986).

Some of these causes are interrelated and some are mutually reinforcing: selective population loss for example may be a contributory factor (via decreased demand) in the demise of companies in the inner cities, but it may also be a reaction to company closures. However, taken together, they present a picture that is rather more complex than just the collapse of inner city economies. The causes of inner city decay are more likely to be multivariate and, whilst it is possible that the collapse of inner city economies would be a contributory factor, it is unlikely that it is the whole story.

We shall subject the idea of an inner city economy to closer scrutiny in Chapter 9 but there are two further considerations consequent upon it and relevant to the logic of the enterprise strategy that should be mentioned here. These will be subjected to more critical treatment in subsequent chapters. The first is a necessary correlate of the notion of an inner city economy and provides a *sine qua non* of the regeneration strategy. It is that there is something *to be* regenerated and that it can be regenerated. It implies the existence of some residual infrastructure which can, by a process of historical reversal, be rejuvenated. This is not to suggest that history can be replicated – technological change alone dictates that the economic bases of inner city economies cannot ever be the same as in their former 'days of glory' – but that some sort of relatively discrete inner city economy can be reconstructed perhaps partly on the basis of manufacturing industries but also on service industries, tourism, high technology and so on. What remains at issue, for the moment at least, is the extent to which such economies would replicate the relatively discrete entities that their antecedents allegedly were: sustaining, and being sustained by the inner city populations. The second – and also related – idea which seems to have achieved canonical status almost by default is that inner city regeneration will only come about by new investment *in* the inner city (however that might be defined). This must of course be necessarily true once the idea of an inner city economy is accepted (supposing – as we do – that such an economy is spatially located in the inner city). That it is an accepted tenet of the enterprise strategy is borne out by current policy practice that directs resources into designated inner city areas (though not all the designated areas, as we shall see, conform to the conventional idea of an inner city area). Now, whilst there is no reason to think that new economic investment in the inner city may not bring some benefit to local populations, it does not follow that this is the only (or the best) strategy. There is an appealing reasonableness to an argument based on spatial discreteness, but it does not follow that investment outwith inner city boundaries (whether designated or not) will not be of benefit to inner city residents. We therefore need to bear in mind that almost all current inner city policy relies heavily on a particular set of assumptions (which are often implicit) about the importance of inner cities as relatively discrete spatial entities. There are possible alternatives and we shall air them when we come to evaluate the logic of the enterprise strategy.

NOTES

1   We shall for present purposes assume 'significant' job creation. Our purpose here is to identify the mechanisms by which the enterprise strategy might have

an effect on deprivation. The *magnitude* of that effect will depend on the level of job creation which is an empirical matter that we cover in subsequent chapters.

2   'Sometimes' because some evidence points to the relative *absence* of spatial overlap between deprivations. This is examined later in this and in subsequent chapters.

3   Confusingly, and often in contravention of the ecological fallacy (Robinson 1950), the term 'multiple deprivation' is often used to denote both these forms of concatenation of different manifestations of deprivation.

4   Some would argue that it is a constant presence, especially in the form of harassment, for ethnic minorities; see Pryce 1979; Kettle and Hodges 1982; Benyon and Solomos 1987; Rex 1988.

5   See, for example, Smith and Squire 1986; Balchin and Bull 1987; Ridge and Smith 1990; Hills and Sutherland 1991.

6   Trickle effect seems to exercise Archbishops of Canterbury. The present Archbishop, Dr George Carey, pointed to its unsatisfactory nature in his maiden speech in the House of Lords (23 May 1991).

5 Trafford Park: Manchester's economic larder

The designation of Trafford Park Development Corporation in February 1987 was a much more instrumental affair than that of the London Docklands six years earlier. If the Docklands had been a grand strategy (the enterprise solution) looking for an area, Trafford Park was more akin to an area looking for a strategy, and what needed to be done seemed tailor-made for the ministrations of the instrument of a development corporation. In this it was more typical of the second generation development corporations (of which it was one) in which corporation status was used more instrumentally than (as was seemingly the case in London and Merseyside) to prove a point.

The Trafford Park Development Corporation (Area and Constitution) Order 1986 was made in December of that year and the Corporation came into being in February 1987 with a life of ten years. The Order designated as the Corporation's urban development area one large plot of land of some 3,000 acres, approximately coterminous with the boundaries of the Trafford Park Industrial Estate, and a second small plot some four miles away in Irlam. The purpose of the designation was quite simply, as the 1980 Local Government Planning and Land Act stipulates, to regenerate the area, in this case the Trafford Park Industrial Estate, which had been in decline both physically and in terms of the number of jobs it provided since the end of the Second World War.

There is of course no such thing as a 'typical' urban development corporation but Trafford is none the less peculiar in a number of respects. Firstly, it is in a location that is crowded with 'inner city' initiatives (see Map 5.1). Parts of both the Trafford and the Salford enterprise zones lie within its boundaries. It abuts the Manchester–Salford Partnership area. It now has another urban development corporation (Central Manchester) on its doorstep, as well as a city action team and the Moss Side/Hulme Task Force.

Secondly, it is, to all intents and purposes, a ready-made site and one that is still economically active (albeit not on the scale that it once was). At the

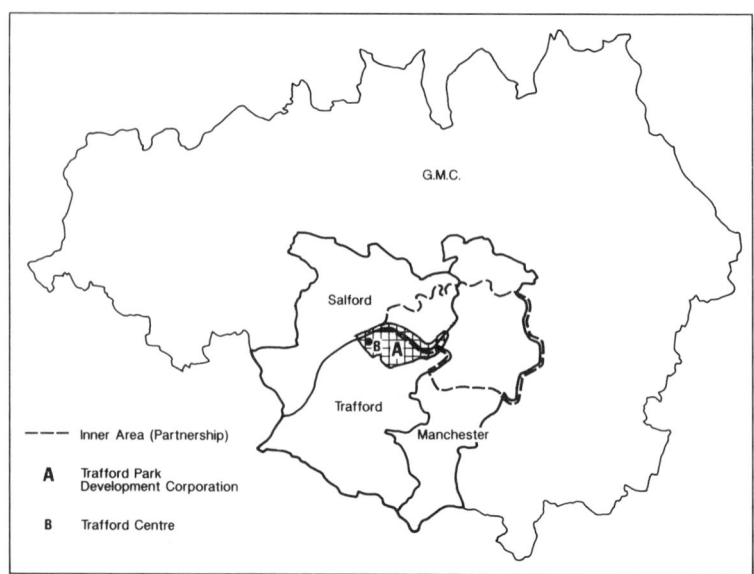

Map 5.1 Trafford Park Development Corporation and Trafford Centre location

time of designation, there were still some 600 companies in the Park including CIBA-Geigy, Kelloggs, GEC, Procter and Gamble and ICI, employing some 24,500 people. Indeed, it was from among such companies as these working jointly with Trafford Council that the impetus came for something to be done about restoring the Park to something like its economic glory in the 1940s.

Thirdly, and most importantly from our point of view, no one lives there. (At designation, forty people were enumerated as living in the Park and there are no more now.) On the face of it therefore, it is an odd place to spearhead inner city regeneration. Why regenerate an area with no population, and who is going to benefit from it? The question opens a debate that we shall enter in more detail in subsequent chapters and is one that concerns definitions of the inner city and whether economic regeneration has to occur *in* residential inner city areas to be of benefit to them. Locationally of course, Trafford Park is surrounded by run-down residential inner city areas and in 1987 there were in excess of 45,000 unemployed within a five-mile radius of it. According to the logic of the 'enterprise solution' therefore (see Chapter 4), substantial new job creation that significantly reduces surrounding inner city unemployment rates will produce trickle down benefits to inner city residents. In theory therefore, and if successful, Trafford Park could become (indeed, in the eyes of its Chief Executive, it has already become) the economic provisioner for the inner areas of Manchester, Trafford and Salford, and it is on this assumption and against this reasoning that we shall evaluate it.

It is interesting therefore that in the past year or two the corporation's relationship with its inner city hinterland has assumed a more prominent place in its publicity material in much the same way that the LDDC has found it necessary to adopt a more accommodating stance to two at least of its overlapping local authorities (and they to it) and to acknowledge that economic regeneration cannot constitute the be-all and end-all of its *raison d'être* and that there must be other ends to be achieved as well. A year after its designation, the Chief Executive of the Trafford Park Development Corporation wrote: 'The Trafford Park UDC is concerned to regenerate a very large run-down industrial estate. It is not responsible for dealing with the complex social problems of the Manchester–Salford Partnership Area' (Shields 1988).

Although the third of the corporation's three specific objectives, first codified in 1988, was 'the translation of the benefits of the economic activity to the local community' (Trafford Park Development Corporation 1988a) attention to how this might be done, and what the local community was, took second place to the promotion of economic growth *per se* at least until about 1990, when the corporation 'designated' eight wards around its perimeter in Manchester, Salford and Trafford as 'priority areas', selected on the basis of unemployment rates and within which the effects of its job creation efforts would be monitored. Four of these wards fall within the area of the Manchester–Salford Partnership.

Perhaps it is in the nature of these 'single-minded authorities' that they have first to convince themselves by their own rhetoric of their single-mindedness, only subsequently to come to the more considered view that this is not an end in itself.

1 A LITTLE HISTORY

Two years after the Manchester Ship Canal was completed in 1894, the de Trafford family began to develop the world's first, and for many years largest, purpose-'built' industrial estate on 1,200 acres of land that it owned alongside the canal. The 'Park' was laid out with networks of roads and railway lines and 600 houses for workers were provided along with shops, near to factory sites. Within five years, forty firms had located in the Park and over the next few years such names as Ford, Westinghouse, Brooke Bond, Rolls-Royce and Guinness were established there (Trafford Park Development Corporation, 1989a, 1990a). Within two decades the Park had become the 'workshop of Manchester' and because of its pre-eminent position was able to weather the depression (in 1935 there were still more than 33,000 people working there). Activity and employment burgeoned between 1939 and 1945 with the wartime effort and the work-force of the Park reached an all-time high during the period of 75,000. The post-war history of the Park however is a familiar one: Trafford Park was like a microcosm of the British manufacturing economy. New technologies replaced traditional manufacturing, and the canal ceased to be a major transportation route. The impact was cumulative: as companies left or died, nothing was done to repair (or at least minimise) the environmental damage, and in consequence the entire Park took on an air of dereliction further undermining any residual confidence that there may have been in it as an entity.

Some big names stayed on, however, and it was one or two of these that responded to Trafford Council's initiative to get something done about the Park as a whole. It is worth noting however that during the 1950s and 1960s, as the Park visibly declined around them, the remaining companies did nothing to minimise the environmental impact (a *confidence*, not a *green* matter in those days); there just was not the mechanism for it to be done. The private sector, unorganised and unsubsidised, could or would do nothing, at least until the mid-1970s. It was from the public sector mainly in the form of Trafford Council that the impetus came. Enterprise had not shown itself to be very enterprising.

The first but not very effective step towards renovating the Park came in 1971 with the formation of the Trafford Park Industrial Council, consisting of a number of companies in the Park, the general aims of which were the promotion of the Park as an industrial and commercial centre and whose immediate concern was environmental improvement (Trafford Park Industrial Council 1990: 1). Little happened however for another decade, when the groundwork was begun for a serious attempt at renewing the Park's infrastructure. By 1983/84, Trafford Council was spending some £1.5m *per annum* on Trafford Park, but this too was proving to be inadequate. The first real advance came during the same year when the Council succeeded in getting the boundaries of the surrounding Assisted Area altered to take in Trafford Park. However, this was only to be a holding operation whilst bigger designs were developed in the shape of a working group consisting of nine major manufacturers in the Park (with the lead role taken by GEC) and representatives of Trafford Council. This group effectively lobbied ministers from the Departments of Environment and Trade and Industry whose response (after a visit to the Park) was that a detailed economic strategy should be drawn up. The working group duly retained five consultancy firms to carry out the task and it is a measure of the degree of government support at this stage that both departments contributed £25,000 each to the costs of the study with Trafford Council and the group of nine companies each contributing another £25,000 (details provided by the Chief Executive of TPDC in an interview; see also Trafford Park Development Corporation 1988b, 1988c).

The Trafford Park Investment Strategy, titulary commissioned jointly by Trafford Park Major Manufacturers, Trafford Metropolitan Borough Council and the Departments of the Environment and Trade and Industry, was published in its final form in 1986 (Trafford Park Investment Strategy 1986). It was a lengthy and detailed document but the nub lay, so far as our story goes, in the three organisational options it proposed to put the strategy into effect. One of these (the report's preferred option) was 'a special type of Urban Development Corporation' (Trafford Park Investment Strategy 1986: 2). Three months after the report emerged, the Trafford Park Development Corporation (Area and Constitution) Order was made.

Whether or not the TPIS report provided the *post hoc* rationale for a decision effectively already made remains open to debate, but it is certainly the case that the effective partnership between Trafford and the private sector, and the willingness (despite a hung council) on the part of most members to hand the Park over to a development corporation, predisposed Conservative ministers to agree to the designation (*Independent*, 5 May 1987).

2 THE ORGANISATION

Like all other urban development corporations, the policy-making arm of TPDC is its Board, comprising eight part-time members 'who have an interest or expertise in aspects of urban regeneration' (Trafford Park Development Corporation 1990b). The Chairman of the Board until 1990 was Peter Hadfield, previously at Bass North West Ltd, and on his retirement the reins were taken over after a seven-month gap by Mr Bill Morgan, formerly of AMEC plc. Leaders of both the Conservative and Labour groups on Trafford Borough Council are among the eight, as is the Deputy Leader of Salford City Council. The number of staff is small at fifty-one, spread over four directorates. Much of the work of the corporation is therefore carried out by outside consultants, expertise being brought-in as and when necessary.

Whilst these arrangements are fairly common amongst development corporations, Trafford is somewhat unusual in that having acquired, by statute, development planning powers for those areas of Salford and Trafford that fall within its boundaries, it now uses the planning departments of both authorities as its agents. It is an arrangement that, until recently at least, could not have been envisaged as practicable in London

Docklands and is a further indication of the preparedness of the two authorities to work in cooperation with the corporation.

3   STRATEGIES

Not surprisingly, the TPIS provided a framework for a strategy for the fledgling Development Corporation, and the Corporate Plan or Mission Statement which sets out the objectives draws heavily on it although it remains fairly skeletal when compared with the original. The Mission Statement itself is extracted from the Local Government Planning and Land Act 1980: 'To secure the physical and economic regeneration of the area' (Trafford Park Development Corporation 1988a: para 1). There follow three objectives:

i)   The generation of increased economic activity and employment through inward and indigenous investment.

ii)   The creation of the highest quality physical environment appropriate to particular types and locations of development, including the provision of a comprehensive range of support services, and marketing and promotion of the area to improve radically its image, and to realise the many opportunities for economic activity which the development area presents.

iii)   The translation of the benefits of the economic activity to the local community.

(Trafford Park Development Corporation 1988a: para 2)

These three objectives are then translated into a strategy consisting of twelve programme areas.

In practice however the energies of the development corporation were put behind some of these objectives (and consequent programmes) to a greater extent than others and for the first three years of its life we can identify three main areas of activity which correspond only in part with the contents of the corporate plan. These were the renewal, replacement and modernisation of the infrastructure and environment of the Park, including improved transport arrangements within and to it. Secondly, there was economic regeneration to be pursued by helping firms already in the Park and attracting new ones from outside. And thirdly, a component of objective (ii), and in essence, a means to the second area of activity above, there was the selling of a new image for the Park. We shall look briefly at these three areas in turn.

Infrastructure

Of the total allocation to TPDC of £160m over ten years, half has been devoted to highways improvement both in and outside the Park (Trafford Park Development Corporation 1990c). Infrastructural improvements were seen at an early stage as the key to attracting economic investment. The Park was, by general consent, environmentally tacky, difficult to get to and difficult to get around once there.

The main road improvements based on a three-spoke highways strategy were to be 'City Link', a new dual carriageway linking the centre of Manchester to the eastern end of the Park (Trafford Park Development Corporation 1989c), a new northerly route out of the Park across the Manchester Ship Canal (the Parkway–M602 Link) giving better access for the more than 50 per cent of the work-force at the Park who live north of the canal (Trafford Park Development Corporation 1989d); and a new southerly route linking Parkway with the M63 (see Map 5.2). In addition, there was to be a new network of 12.5 miles of internal primary, secondary and local roads (Trafford Park Development Corporation 1988b: 6).[1]

The other proposed transportation investment (supported by TPDC but in fact a Greater Manchester Passenger Transport Executive Scheme) was Metrolink or a light rapid transit (a small railway) branching off the planned route from Bury to Altrincham into the Park and on (in the more optimistic version) through the Park to Dumplington at the far western end (see Kirby 1988). The cost was roughly calculated in 1988 at £20m to reach the centre of the Park, and more if it went to Dumplington. However, it was anticipated that most of the funding would come from the private sector. It was hoped to have the first phase in operation by 1992. As of 1991 however, it seemed more likely that if it happens at all it will not be within the lifetime of the development corporation. But more of that later.

Economic development

With no detailed design, the attraction of businesses into the area was always going to be opportunistic and always with the hope of the 'big catch'. Preferred users would be high technology, science parks, light industrial, office and commercial and retail and leisure, as well as manufacturing which had always been the staple of the Park. And the search for investors would concentrate on the south of England, the USA, and, to a lesser extent, Europe (Trafford Park Development Corporation 1988a: 2).

Coupled with the attraction of new investment to the Park would be assistance to companies already there, to compete effectively and, where possible and desired, to expand. What the corporation wanted to avoid was

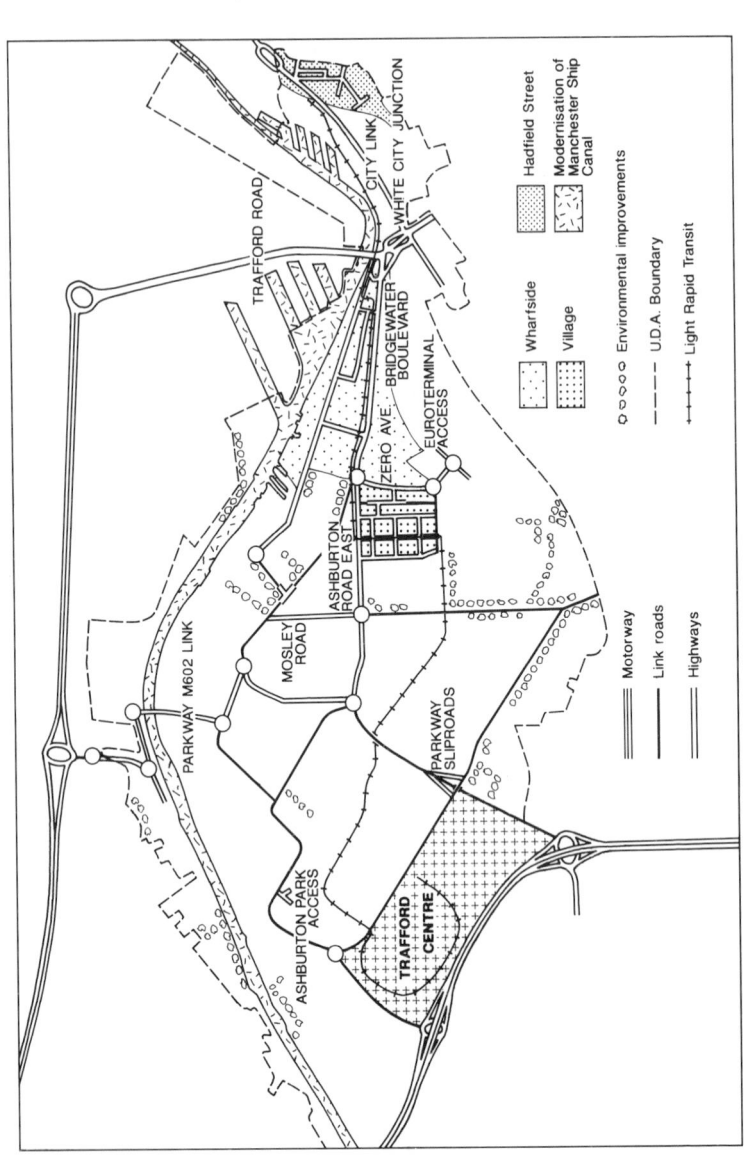

Map 5.2 Trafford Park Development Corporation main programme areas

to have inward investment-gain offset by closures or exodus of existing companies.

By 1991 some sixteen developments were under way, though some are still in the planning stage. Two of these in particular stand out for their ambitiousness however: the Exchange Quay development in the Salford Enterprise Zone and the Wharfside area at the eastern end of the Park within which one large speculative development – the Quay West Office block – has been completed (and was opened in May 1991).

In one sense, the investment strategy has been hampered by what might have appeared to have been a bonus. There are six enterprise zones in the proximity of the Park (the three Trafford and three Salford enterprise zones) and parts of some of these overlap with the corporation's designated area. As the original TPIS strategy predicted, these have proved to be more attractive with the higher levels of subsidy they could offer, and this had blighted demand in the surrounding Park even before the corporation was designated. And so it has continued to be. Progress towards a self-sustaining regeneration of the *whole* Park may turn out to be a flawed strategy so long as more powerful magnets remain outside or within small parts of it (though it should be noted that the enterprise zones came to an end in August 1991).

Selling a new image

The TPIS set great store by the creation of a new image for Trafford Park:

> Central to the concept of the physical proposals for Trafford Park is the creation of a new image and the impression of a completely different and far better environment. This will require coordinated overall policies with attention to priority areas to achieve the maximum early impact and thereby stimulate investment.
>
> (Trafford Park Investment Strategy 1986: 39)

The corporation took this injunction on board and one of the first things it undertook was a two-year (but now still continuing) 'awareness campaign' to create and sell a new image for the Park. To begin with of course, there was little to sell other than visions and its own confidence – and such assets as could be mustered from the location of the Park near to Manchester, and close to a large labour force.

There is no reason to think that the confidence on sale was manufactured – it is something that the enterprise culture is not short of – even if at times excitement gets the better of judgement and results in some hyperbole. Nor is there reason to believe that this was anything but the right strategy to adopt. After all, the TPIS analysis had identified the run-down and negative image of the Park as one of, if not the, main stumbling blocks to revival. And if Trafford Park was to be sold around the world it had to be sold as somewhere that investors could have confidence in. Thus the then Chairman of the Board, Peter Hadfield, interviewed for a local newspaper, commented: 'We hope it will become the crown of the north west, not only in industrial terms but also as a residential and leisure centre.'

Again, a typical sales pitch reads: 'Here at Trafford Park we have initiated a multi-million pound re-development project for a new and prosperous tomorrow. And we are supremely confident in what we offer' (Trafford Park Development Corporation 1990c). Ministers had also learned their lines. Mr David Trippier, having donned the obligatory hard hat to visit the site of the new Quay West development in 1988, opined that 'This development illustrates the confidence which the private sector now has in the future of the inner cities and, in particular, in the urban development areas' (Trippier 1988).

Apart from confidence, there have also been the infrastructure arrangements and subsidies to sell and – for potential migrant firms from outside the north west – the Hallé Orchestra, the Royal Exchange Theatre, the Opera House, the Lake District and Snowdonia (Trafford Park Development Corporation 1990a). And a work-force of over one million within easy reach 'of an unusually high calibre and. . .keen to work. . .and to obtain new skills'.

However, if the development corporation does not have to worry too much about Snowdonia or the Hallé, it does have to stump up the infrastructure it has promised if migrant and potentially migrant companies are to maintain their confidence and fulfil their commitment to invest. But as we shall subsequently see, some promises may be too ambitious to fulfil, and grandiose claims made in the exuberance of the early years may begin to look like embarrassments.

Job creation and training

If, in the earlier years, job creation was not promoted by the corporation as a key aim of the enterprise, it could perhaps justifiably argue that it was a necessary and automatic concomitant of economic regeneration. Of course jobs would be created by the regeneration process; the only uncertainties might be how many and of what kind (although the 'how many' was soon answered by adopting the figure of 16,000 from the TPIS strategy). However, the London Docklands experience had by then shown that perhaps the single area of urban development corporations' activities most vulnerable to attack was the adequacy or otherwise of the benefits accruing to the local communities. Increasingly therefore, TPDC came to assert the importance of local benefit by ensuring that the jobs created went, so far as possible, to local people and that adequate training facilities were provided for those who needed skills enhancement. Thus, the Deputy Chairman, in the corporation's Annual Report for 1989–90, claimed that 'The creation of lasting jobs in our area is a central objective in the Corporation's task of economic regeneration' (Trafford Park Development Corporation 1990b: 3). And again, the Foreword to the TPDC Labour Market Survey of 1989 argued that within the broad strategy of economic and physical regeneration 'the Corporation is committed to ensuring that the resulting increased economic activity should benefit the local community. To further this aim the Corporation has established an employment and training team' (Trafford Park Development Corporation 1989e).

As additional focus to its 'community benefit' strategy, the development corporation has, whenever possible, encouraged developers to use local building companies for construction work, and expanding or inwardly migrating firms to employ local labour. (Communication from Publicity Manager, Trafford Park Development Corporation, 1991.) The 'local community' is then specified as Trafford, Salford and parts of Manchester (and not just the eight priority area wards noted above). No data are available to enable a judgement to be made about whether this 'encouragement' has produced the desirable results and, so far as we are aware, none have been collected.

Any job creation forecast will of course be highly speculative and the TPIS strategy figure of 16,000 (now enshrined in a number of TPDC documents) was no doubt as good as any other at the time (and much hangs, as we shall subsequently see, on what counts as a 'new job'). But as a benchmark for performance measurement purposes, it is probably of little value, especially in the light of forecasts, for particular developments within the park – from 6,000 to 10,000 for the Wharfside development, and 3,000 to 4,000 for the Northbank Estate at Irlam (the separate small development area). If Wharfside were to produce 10,000 and Northbank 4,000 jobs, only another 2,000 jobs would be required over the whole of the remainder of the Park in order to reach the adopted TPIS figure. It is probably best therefore to treat most of these as figures plucked from the air. They don't add up and have little value as strategic indicators.

There are a variety of ways of increasing the chances of the local labour force (and particularly the unemployed) getting the newly created jobs, and in the absence of any local labour contracts (which could only be voluntary and unenforceable), probably the best way is to ensure by various forms of training that the skills of the labour force match those required by the new jobs. (We shall examine *how* effective such a strategy is in a later chapter.)

The organisation and provision of training is the responsibility of the training and employment team. The team has developed four types of training scheme which are provided by local education institutions and are subsidised in various degrees by the corporation.

Job Offer Training (JOT) is available to companies that have vacancies and where an unemployed candidate can be trained in the particular skills for the job. The corporation will pay 75 per cent of the costs of the training on condition of the guarantee of a job (details from an interview with Mr K. Turner, Employment and Training Manager; see also Trafford Park Development Corporation 1990e; Southern 1990).

Extra Skills Training (EST) is intended to exploit the 'stepladder' approach to employment provision by providing additional skills training for people already in employment so that they can move up the skills hierarchy thus vacating a position for a currently unemployed person with fewer skills.

Customised Training (CT) requires that a company undergoing expansion makes a commitment to employ a certain number of locally unemployed people. In return, the development corporation will provide pre-interview training and confidence-building, and if the candidate passes the selection process it will part-finance training in the particular skills the company requires.

The fourth scheme, 'Workout', is designed to offer young job applicants help and advice in making job applications, telephone and interview techniques and in self presentation. Again, the scheme, run in cooperation with Salford City Council, is part-funded by the corporation.

Participation, consultation and accountability

Of the variety of levels of consultation and participation in decision making, it is the involvement of the local community that is the most problematic for TPDC. Local community participation of course became a running sore for the London Docklands Corporation and that experience clearly suggested that a development corporation ignores the local community at its peril. Trafford Park's problem is that there is no obvious local community either to consult or to ignore. The Park has no indigenous population to speak of (forty at designation) and there is no evidence that people living in areas around it have any proprietorial sense towards it. Certainly, there has been none of the vociferous (and sometimes effective) opposition to the activities of the corporation that have been a feature of the London Docklands. Nor, as we have noted, did the corporation, as a 'single-minded body', appear particularly concerned in its early days with the impact of its activities within the urban development area or other areas outwith the boundary. After this initial phase of getting the operation moving, a greater concern with consulting the 'local community' emerged, but the problem remained of who, or what, could realistically fill this role. In consequence, a number of 'communities' has emerged, the two principal ones being surrounding residential areas (in effect Trafford, Salford and the more proximate parts of Manchester), and businesses located within the Park. In the latter case, however, it remains unclear whether it is the interests of the businesses themselves or of their employees that are salient. Nor would it be reasonable to anticipate that those in the Park's residential orbit will have a community of interest towards it. The impact of the development corporation's activities for example may well be very different as between those who view and use it as an employment source, and those upon whom its impact is primarily or solely environmental. It will therefore matter *which* of the Park's 'local communities' is consulted.

None the less, the somewhat amorphous nature of its constituencies has not prevented the corporation from stressing the importance of consultation (but not, explicitly at least, participation) or of setting up the machinery to effect it. This is what the Chairman of the Board had to say about the consultation procedure:

> The Corporation is very conscious of the need to involve the local community in all its planning and decision making. So we have conducted a programme of public consultation, with explanatory brochures, public briefings, a free-phone hotline and one-to-one meetings as necessary between all interested parties and the Corporation's staff and consultants.

> (Hadfield 1988)

Since then, the corporation has developed five principal means of consulting and informing communities in its hinterland: a community liaison committee, two 'community' papers (*Profile* and *Link-Up*), by links with established community groups and by contacts with companies (largely at senior management level).

The most ambitious and significant of these mechanisms is the Community Liaison Committee chaired by a member of the corporation's Board, and made up of two members of the corporation staff (the Chief Executive and the Employment and Training Manager), and representatives of Salford, Trafford and Manchester local authorities (at member level), trade councils, the churches, the Moss Side Community Development Trust (representing a number of community groups in Moss Side), the Village Traders Association, the Enterprise Agency, the Groundwork Trust, the trade unions and other business interests. Meetings of this committee (every two months) and the production of associated public briefing documents for use at public meetings now constitute probably the primary form of consultation with the local communities. However, this is consultation rather than participation. The views of the Community Liaison Committee on the activities of the corporation are 'reported to, and considered by, the Board and weighed carefully in the decision-making process' (Annual Report 1990), but they remain an input to this process and the committee takes no part in decision making itself.

None the less, the views of the committee and opinions expressed in reaction to public briefing documents at public meetings have had some impact, if only marginal, on some decisions. Some of the main consultation exercises involving the production of 'public briefing' documents have been in connection with several of the developments already referred to – the City Link, Wharfside, the Parkway–M602 link and the Northbank Industrial Estate at Irlam. One other concerned the redevelopment of the 'village' – a small enclave of shops and (originally) housing within the Park. As might be expected, the briefing papers for the highways proposals present alternative routings for the new roads, and views on the most suitable are invited. The briefing documents for Wharfside, the Northbank estate and the Village, however, are speculative and contain no alternative sets of proposals to comment on or choose between and in this respect they hardly constitute 'consultation' documents. Evidence of the nature of the consultation procedures therefore, and what they have produced, is scarce. The claim in the Annual Report for 1990, that the Community Liaison Committee had been 'instrumental in determining the routes of the new bus services into Trafford Park', does not impress with the centrality of the influence of the committee. Only in respect of the Village does community input (though which community it is not clear) appear to have had significant results – though here again, only at the level of 'ideas which (the corporation) intend to pursue'. These ideas included a change in the balance between manufacturing and office/high-technology use; the provision of a crèche–nursery; a higher priority for the provision of security systems, and the refurbishing of the existing Trafford Park Hotel to a middle, rather than high price range hotel (Trafford Park Development Corporation 1990e).

Besides consultation with the local communities, the corporation has of course to work alongside, and with, two local authorities: Trafford and Salford. Co-ordination and cooperation with these authorities is of vital importance to the effective functioning of the development corporation and this must apply not least to those of its activities which have an impact on the populations of these towns. The corporation is statutorily obliged to consult the two authorities on its planning and strategy decisions but it is fair to say that it views its relations with them as a good deal closer than statutory consultation: 'The role of this Development Corporation is characterised by partnership. We will continue to work hard to maintain our excellent relations with the Borough of Trafford and the City of Salford' (Shields 1990).

There is a good deal of substance to this claim. Indeed, there is no reason to doubt that the corporation has observed to the full the detailed requirements stipulated in the Consultation Code, which lays out the form of consultation and the duties of the corporation in this respect (Trafford Park Development Corporation 1988d). Cooperation takes place at a number of levels from the Board of the corporation, almost half the membership of which is made up of local authority councillors, to day-to-day activity at the departmental level particularly in the field of training. And as we have already noted, the planning departments of the two authorities act as agents for the development corporation.

There appears therefore to have been none of the animosity between the development corporation and overlapping local authorities that so characterised the formative (and middle) years of the London Docklands Development Corporation, and this is no doubt due in large measure to the involvement of Trafford in attracting development corporation status for the Park.

The Community Initiatives Programme

Like other development corporations, Trafford Park does not have responsibilities that extend to social provision, but it does have an obligation (it is the third of its objectives in the corporate plan) to ensure that some, at least, of the benefits of regeneration flow to local communities. The principal means by which the corporation pursues this objective is through its Community Initiatives Programme. Before outlining the substance of this programme however, it is worth saying something about what the corporation does *not* do. We have argued that the logic of the enterprise strategy dictates that benefit to local communities will come as a result of the job growth that attends regeneration. The unemployed will become employed and the benefits of this will trickle down to the dependent population. If this is not the case, we should not pretend that the enterprise strategy is inner city strategy. And if local benefit is not a necessary causal consequence of economic regeneration then anything that local communities get out of it will look like inconsequential hand-outs. It cannot be over-emphasised that the purpose of the enterprise strategy is to set in motion an economic process, a necessary and constitutive part of which is benefit to local people. It is not (and here we are assuming the guise of its proponents) intended to produce hand-outs for the deprived. Much therefore hinges on local people getting the jobs and part of the strategy must (presumably) be to maximise the chances of this happening. The Trafford Park Development Corporation has not pursued a robust policy of *maximising* local benefit in this way. What it has done is to institute a Community Initiatives Programme, the substance of which we can now outline.

There are twenty-three items in the Programme as at June 1991. We list them all below in summary form:

- consultation (including the Community Liaison Committee)
- involvement with, and support for, Manchester TEC
- redundancy counselling services
- publicity campaign on employment and training assistance
- governors of local schools and education/industry links
- grants to voluntary bodies (up to £250 per grant)
- job offer training scheme
- joint founder of Trafford Education Business Partnership
- support for Salford Compact and the Salford Education Business Partnership
- provision of IT equipment to fifty-two local schools
- support for pre-vocational training
- ability to devise customised training packages
- extra skills training
- provision of computer equipment for the partially disabled
- circulation of *Link-Up* (community newspaper)
- possibility of corporation's construction projects being used for job training
- Job Club for 16–19 year olds
- development of further training schemes and aid to businesses
- funding support for Business Watch (security scheme)
- developing other security schemes for business
- support for Trafford Park Arts in Industry Committee
- possible support for energy-efficient initiatives
- clerical/computer and administration training for ethnic minority women.

(Trafford Park Development Corporation 1991a)

The list (expenditure on the items in which was £417,000 at May 1991) appears to include all activities undertaken by the corporation other than infrastructure works and business promotion – a sort of catch-all category. The largest single component on the list consists of projects to help local people obtain employment by way of the provision or promotion of various types of training (some ten items, several of which have already been noted). They do not, however, despite their variety, add up to a robust strategy for the promotion of training on a large scale.

When training schemes are taken out, the remainder of the list consists largely of consultation exercises, links between schools and business, the provision of grants and equipment and security schemes for business.

4 PROGRESS AND ACHIEVEMENTS

The Trafford Park Development Corporation is only five years old at the time of writing and any assessment of its achievements can only be preliminary. None the less, it is possible after this time to note what has been done and whether the enterprise appears to be on course. The early years of a development corporation must necessarily be devoted to planning and preparing the groundwork. The substance of what they are about – the concrete and glass and the jobs (and the alleviation of deprivation lest that be forgotten) must come later as they move towards the twilight of their years. Trafford Park is just at the point when the years of preparation turn into the years of delivery. That, at any rate, is the assessment of its Chief Executive: 'the next twelve months will see. . .changes after four years of digging the foundations of success' (Shields 1991).

It is therefore worth bearing in mind that progress is not linear and that if TPDC is now approaching the mid point of its planned life, we should not necessarily expect to see 40 per cent of its total anticipated output. None the less, the strategies that we outlined earlier should by now be yielding some tangible results. Such as these are, we summarise in this section.

Firstly, however, tables 5.1 and 5.2 provide selected summary data of progress to April 1991. These data and the review of progress that follows will provide evidence for our evaluations in Chapters 9 and 10.

Infrastructure

Probably the most time-consuming part of new road developments is obtaining the necessary compulsory purchase orders (CPOs) for land along the route. So it is with the Parkway/M602 link (see page 79). The route of the link has been agreed and the public inquiry in connection with the necessary CPOs took place in April 1991, and construction began in the Summer of 1992 (Trafford Park Development Corporation 1991b). The second major scheme to link the park with the centre of Manchester (City Link) has been taken over by Trafford MBC with the Department of Transport. The third (eastern spine) radial route was to be subject to CPO hearings during 1991. However, the important Trafford Wharf Road which feeds the Wharfside development is now under reconstruction. All the other road schemes remain at the design stage at the time of writing.

The other major transportation strategy – the extension into the Park of the Light Rapid Transit railway – has not progressed; no commitment of private sector funding has been forthcoming, and it now seems unlikely that this will be constructed before the end of the life of the development corporation. Although the railway is a responsibility of the Greater Manchester

Table 5.1 Trafford Park: achievements in four programme areas and in UDA as a whole

| Programme Area | TPDC Expenditure (£000s) | Land Reclaimed (ha) | Outputs | | | |
			Development (m²)	New Jobs	Private Sector Investment (£000s)	Infrastructure (km)
Village	4,042	2.64	420	0	128	0
Irlam	11,309	15.01	5,380	177	2,135	1.9
Hadfield Street	2,288	0.30	2,800	52	783	0
Wharfside	9,063	3.88	5,313	151	1,678	0.58
Total – UDA	69,467	61.28	209,900 (2.26m sq ft)	3,517	490,000	4.28

Source: Trafford Park Development Corporation, *Key Statistics, May 1991*

Table 5.2 Trafford Park: Environmental and other achievements

Environmental
- over 100 schemes completed or under way
- £9m expenditure to date
- approximately 10,000 trees planted
- 18,000m² of new cladding or recladding
- 9 km of new or improved fencing/walls/railings

Other
- 16 major developments completed or under way
- 129.08 hectares of land in TPDC ownership
- over 3,000 business enquiries dealt with
- 359 planning applications determined

Source: Trafford Park Development Corporation, *Key Statistics, May 1991*

Passenger Transport Executive it will, if it does not go ahead, seriously compromise the chances of self-sustaining regeneration in the Park.

Economic development

We have noted elsewhere that the 'gearing ratio' or 'leverage' is often seen (not least by government) as the key diagnostic of the health of a development corporation. But gearing ratios are slippery animals and will depend at any given time on the amount the corporation has spent and how much private sector investment has been committed. The balance between the two will necessarily continue to shift.

As of April 1991 the Trafford Park Development Corporation had spent £68m and had attracted £490m of private sector investment, giving a gearing ratio of 7:1 (Communication from Publicity Manager, Trafford Park Development Corporation 1991). This is less than some of the estimates for LDDC in its halcyon days (see Chapter 6) and probably higher than the final out-turn ratio. However, TPDC had bought itself more leverage power by increasing its initial grant from the government of £160m to £200m by land sales. Whether more leverage money can produce a higher final gearing ratio only time will tell.

There has been a net increase of 300 companies in the Park since 1987, but as the rate of start-up and closure or migration of small firms had been high it is not possible to say what sort of gross movements have produced this net figure.

Of the two most ambitious developments in the Park that we noted earlier, Wharfside has been the subject of a revised master plan in which the area to be developed in the immediate future has been much reduced in size and the grandiose scheme for comprehensive development has been replaced 'on a phased basis at a pace which reflects market conditions' (Trafford Park Development Corporation 1991b). What this means is that the pace will be both slower and more cautious. Wharfside has not gone well and the initial plan was probably too ambitious to survive the recession undamaged. There is, as we have seen, one completed office block, Quay West, developed by the property arm of the Manchester Ship Canal Company but this has remained without prospective tenants for some time, an imposing pink glass edifice in a sea of dereliction, and with a hopelessly inadequate and poor quality road system to serve it (though as noted above, work has now begun on Trafford Wharf Road).

Wharfside and Quay West amply demonstrate the problem of timing for a development corporation. In the heady days at the end of the last decade, the corporation was promising infrastructure works which, in the event, it could not provide – at least not in time to maximise the profitability of Quay West. If a development corporation cannot deliver the infrastructure services for investment capital (for whatever reason, and having given the impression that it could), then the private sector is likely to adopt a more cautious approach in its investment plans, notwithstanding the other financial attractions. The revised plan for Wharfside recognises this difficulty and work is progressing both on environmental improvements and improved roads.

The second 'grand scheme' – the Exchange Quay development by Charter Developments – is still under construction and on target and will provide 500,000 square feet of office space with associated shops and services. This makes it the single largest office development in the north west, and possibly outside London. The prognosis is healthier than for Quay West (with which it is in competition) with most of the buildings already sold.

A number of other schemes are progressing more or less on schedule at Pomona Strand and Water's Edge (office developments), Centrepoint and Northbank (Irlam) industrial estates and the Empress Business Centre in the Hadfield Street Industrial Improvement Area. However, there is one other development that deserves comment because it too has suffered slippage. Plans for redeveloping the 'village' at the heart of the Park were drawn up in mid-1989 but there is no visible change other than for some grassing and tree planting. Nor is there likely to be until 1992; the report of the inquiry into the compulsory purchase orders was not due until late Summer 1991. (There were, however, four developers waiting in the wings.) It will therefore be five years from the start of TPDC before any real change is evident in the Village: a long time for a 'single-minded' agency to produce the 'swift impact' that its first Chairman said in 1988 was 'imperative' (Trafford Park Development Corporation 1988b).

Job creation and skills training

As of April 1991 the development corporation estimates that 3,260 new jobs had been created in the Park as a result of companies moving in and of construction work. Unfortunately, no breakdown is available to indicate what sorts of jobs these are, whether they are full- or part-time – and importantly, whether they have gone to 'local' people. Neither is it possible to say how many jobs might have been preserved as a result of the corporation's activities – a figure that might be a significant component in its final balance sheet.

Some forty or so people have been through the various training schemes that the corporation offers and a further 580 places have been assisted, but it is intended that training will now be marketed more aggressively. The Training and Employment Manager offered two reasons why so few people had taken up the possibility of training. The first was a lack of interest on the part of companies moving to the Park for whom work-force availability was often far down their list of priorities. The other was finding unemployed people who could fulfil the requirements for the courses. It is also worth noting that feedback from consultation with the local communities indicated that the provision of jobs and training were not among their major concerns. Physical dereliction and crime appeared to be nearer the front of people's minds.

5   AFTER FOUR YEARS

Trafford Park Development Corporation has been, and is, selling itself hard in this country, in Europe and in the USA. Early claims were however perhaps a little immodest and some of the early schemes too ambitious. But then you have to sell your product to yourself before you can effectively sell it to others. But the early heady days were followed by days of recession and there has had to be some retrenchment. There is sufficient in the pipeline for the moment, but the number and rate of enquiries from companies has fallen back and, in order to maintain momentum, the corporation has targeted companies in the 'M4 corridor' and sent out information and a questionnaire to 16,000 of them. Clearly, it is neither a time nor a situation for sitting back and relaxing.

Meanwhile, there are 300 new companies in Trafford Park, 3,260 new jobs, £490m of private sector investment, but an infrastructure plan that is behind schedule, no LRT in sight and two premier schemes at the Village and Wharfside that are flagging.

NOTE

1   As part of the infrastructural works at Irlam, the small and separate designated area of the corporation, a new £24m bypass of the Northbank estate was also planned.

6 Docklands: Flagship or Titanic?

No evaluation of inner city policy can possibly exclude events in the London Docklands since the area was designated as a development corporation: London Docklands Development Corporation (LDDC) in 1981. The claims made on both sides are simply too extreme to ignore. For the government, the Docklands experiment points the way to the future. In his review of progress on inner city policy in April 1987, John Patten, then Minister of Housing and Construction, commented that

> Radical and direct government action is being focused through the UDCs to tackle problems that the local authorities cannot and/or will not deal with alone and where the private sector has been deterred from investing. The two UDCs so far established, in Merseyside and Docklands have shown how successful this approach can be – in London Dockland spectacularly so.

Patten used this judgement as the basis for some broader conclusions:

> Economic change in our cities and the damage caused by excessive municipal intervention did not happen overnight. Renewal will not be instantaneous either. But well-directed initiatives can achieve a great deal – London Docklands may, with the benefit of 20:20 hindsight look an easy nut to have cracked; it certainly did not look easy before the Development Corporation was established.
>
> (*Guardian*, 17 April 1987)

Action for Cities (1988), the policy document launching the post-election phase of inner city policy, confirmed this judgement, with its fulsome references to Docklands as the prime example of the success of enterprise-led development and complete omission of any reference to local government. Then and subsequently, ministers have lost no opportunity to underline the fundamental significance of the approach adopted. This approach was still being employed – even if in modified form – in the tenth anniversary speech delivered by the politician who was responsible for launching the experiment, Michael Heseltine.

For the government's critics, the lessons are entirely different. The Bishop of Stepney, giving written evidence to the House of Commons Employment Committee (1988), observed that:

> It is my strong impression that the initial and then long-standing difficulties caused by the imposition of the LDDC both brought severe fragmentation and also missed out on the opportunities offered of strategic social reconstruction.
>
> (House of Commons Employment Committee 1988b: 42)

The President of the Royal Town Planning Institute, at a conference in the following year, referred to the Docklands as 'a failure that has been rejected even by its own disciples' (Brownill 1990: 133). His reaction is not unusual. Bob Colenutt, in another recent survey, comments that 'it is no longer fashionable to say anything nice about the LDDC' (Keith and Rogers 1991: 31). The development corporation does still have its outside champions. For example, the sociologist David Marsland, first recipient of the Margaret Thatcher award, recently described the Docklands as 'the most exciting, positive and potentially profitable (in every sense of that maligned word) development in Europe' (Marsland 1991). But the most recent full academic appraisal, Sue Brownill's *Developing London's Docklands*, concludes flatly that the lesson of Docklands is that 'market-led planning does not work' (Brownill 1990: 13). The acute financial difficulties experienced by the developers of Canary Wharf, Olympia & York, early in 1992 reinforced that conclusion.

However, behind Brownill's simple conclusion lies a different and more complex question about the causes of the Docklands' successes and failures. Do these outcomes stem not from the way in which the market has functioned – or failed to do so – but rather from the form of public sector intervention that was adopted? This would certainly be consistent with the way in which Michael Heseltine set out the argument in his triumphalist account of the origins of the development corporations, *Where There's a Will* (Heseltine 1987), with its stress on providing the 'sinews' for renewal, despite Treasury anxieties about 'a wide opening for additional public expenditure'. His critics have made the same point. As Brownill puts it, 'It (the LDDC) does not work on its own terms because it is not market led but dependent on public activity and investment' (Brownhill 1990: 13).

If there is some doubt about whether it is the free market or an alternative form of corporatism that is being tested out in the London Docklands, there can be no question about the high political profile of the initiative and in particular its significance for local government. Claims for the success of the Docklands enterprise reinforce arguments for the exclusion of local authorities from what Batley has called 'central corporatism operated locally'. He goes on:

> In setting up the first UDCs, the Government took the view that existing arrangements involving local authorities were 'inadequate to deal with the complex task of regeneration' (National Audit Office 1988). Does this imply a concern, on the part of Government, to squeeze local government out of its burgeoning role in local economic development and hence out of the realm of corporatist politics?
>
> (Batley 1989: 169)

This interpretation receives some support from a pamphlet published for Aims of Industry by one of the government's prominent supporters among the property developers, Nigel Mobbs of Slough Estates. Under the general rubric of 'public administration', Mobbs criticised local authorities for their 'alien policies and ill-conceived intervention' and argued that 'the party political element should be removed from policy and decision making', where necessary through a wider use of UDCs and 'the temporary deletion of traditional local government boundaries and demarcation' (Mobbs 1986: 11).

Or was there a simpler motive at work – not so much excluding politics as changing them? In an interview conducted while he was still on the backbenches, Michael Heseltine commented of the local authorities affected by the declaration of the UDC:

> These people have created an environment which is wholly unattractive to a balanced society, but then there is no question of them ever controlling it. The politics of the area will change. Once you have a balanced community they won't be able to get away with this nonsense. It's a political and social revolution.
>
> (*Municipal Journal*, 24 October 1986)

A second bone of contention is whether the experience of the London Docklands is unique. The nature of the area and the complex physical layout; its location next to the City of London; the size and composition of the resident population; the precipitate decline of economic activity within the area over the post-war period; and the complex history of past attempts at regeneration and the constellation of relationships that have developed as a result, have all been advanced as reasons why the London Docklands case is special. On the other hand, the powers given to the LDDC and the political and technical characteristics of the approach adopted there are similar to those followed elsewhere, at least in the earlier phases of the Conservatives' inner city policy. Nor are the locational, economic and social issues wholly distinctive. What does chiefly distinguish London Docklands is the high profile that it has enjoyed – its 'flagship' status – which has guaranteed it continued attention as the exemplar of government policy and also the lion's share of resources from public funds (see Table 6.1).

In this sense, despite the special characteristics of both the local and the London situation – and latterly the tendency of other UDCs to distance themselves from the Docklands experience – it is legitimate to use the Docklands as a key test of the effectiveness of the government's inner city policies.

For reasons shortly to be set out in greater detail, an evaluation of the ten years of the LDDC is less straightforward than might be supposed from the multiplicity of claims just quoted (and others). There is no master plan for the corporation's activities. Targets for achievement in different sectors of activity are approximate and subject to sudden revision. On occasion, they seem to be plucked out of the air – witness the Acting Chief Executive's performance when questioned by the House of Commons Employment Committee in April 1988 about rates of unemployment. To the patent astonishment of the Committee, he declared that the corporation's policy objective was to bring the Docklands' unemployment level down below the Greater London average (House of Commons Employment Committee 1988b).

What are referred to as the development corporation's 'corporate plans' have been in essence bids for resource allocation to be negotiated with the

Table 6.1 Grants-in-aid to urban development corporations, 1981–90

UDC	Total (£m)	%
London Docklands	1098.8	59.3
Merseyside	232.8	12.6
Teesside	103.8	5.6
Tyne and Wear	101.6	5.5
Black Country	95.4	5.1
Trafford Park	63.5	3.4
Cardiff Bay	58.8	3.2
Sheffield	36.4	2.0
Leeds	25.5	1.4
Bristol	18.7	1.0
Central Manchester	17.5	0.9

Source: DoE as cited by LDCC

Department of the Environment as the channel for public finds and then used in negotiation with potential investors. Latterly, for reasons that will also be elaborated upon later, there has been a change of approach: substantial new policy documents have been issued in which objectives have been defined more broadly. But although these are described as 'plans', they still fall some way short of what that term is generally supposed to imply.

However, some of this shortfall can be made up from other sources. The London Docklands Consultative Committee (LDCC) – a locally-based lobbying organisation – has produced a series of reviews of the LDDC's activities, at four, six, eight and ten years after declaration. A fuller book-length account of the Docklands experience now exists (Brownill 1990), together with a group of other academic appraisals, accounts by architectural critics of the physical form of the new Docklands and eyewitness descriptions of the impact of the changes on the ground (e.g. Widgery 1991). There is even a new sub-genre of recent novels with Docklands settings. Perhaps not surprisingly, most of these offer a different perspective to that of the LDDC and the numerous consultants that it has employed. From all these sources, a composite portrait can be built up of the corporation as it appeared on reaching its tenth birthday in July 1991 – late middle-age, if its timespan of activity remains fifteen years, as initially intended.

THE NATURE OF THE BEAST

The London Docklands Development Corporation is an urban development corporation set up, like all UDCs, under the Local Government Planning and Land Act 1980. It was one of the first two to be declared, the other being the one on Merseyside and, like all others, its function, as defined in Section 136 of the Act, is to *regenerate* the area for which it is responsible by 'bringing land and buildings into effective use, encouraging the development of existing and new industry and commerce, creating an attractive environment and ensuring that housing and social facilities are available to encourage people to live and work in the area'. To discharge these responsibilities, the development corporation replaces the local authority as development control authority and is given power to have land 'vested' in it by Parliament, with no recourse to appeal. One specific feature of the Docklands situation was the simultaneous creation of an enterprise zone in the Isle of Dogs, with the associated exemptions from tax, rates and controls. The UDC also became the channel for urban programme grants within its area of activity.

The London boroughs within whose area the LDDC was established therefore lost substantially – both in powers and resources – as a result of its establishment. In the event, three boroughs were affected by this loss of control over development and building land: Tower Hamlets, Southwark and Newham. In the earlier phase of activity during the 1970s, when a local authority-based Docklands Joint Committee supervised the preparation and implementation of a London Docklands Strategic Plan, five boroughs along the Thames riverside were included, together with the GLC. On declaration, Greenwich and Lewisham were excluded, but their exclusion did not help to make the area a more coherent entity. The concept of 'Docklands' is intrinsically artificial, if the linking element of the presence of the Docks themselves along both banks of the Thames is excluded. The river forms a natural barrier which is not easily crossed. The relationship of local people is to neighbourhoods – Wapping, Beckton, Isle of Dogs, Poplar, Limehouse, North Southwark – with substantially differing traditions and social and ethnic compositions, although all of them have had in common a predominantly working-class population with a comparatively narrow range of skills and work experience.

The resources initially available to the LDDC included not only land – 6,500 acres were initially vested in the corporation – but a substantial annual grant allocated through the Department of the Environment, on the basis of the corporate plan. This is released scheme by scheme, which permits the DoE to monitor progress: the money can be used for any activity that falls within the scope of Section 136 of the Act. Initially, funds were spent principally on purchase of land and site preparation; the land bank, once established, grew rapidly until by the later 1980s the corporation's earnings from the sale of land to developers began for a while to exceed its subvention from the DoE. This development appeared to give some substance to the claim made by the corporation's first Chief Executive, Reg Ward, who saw the funding pattern as 'maintaining short-term high front-end loading falling sharply to a very low level of ongoing public funding support. . .pump-priming over a relatively short period' (London Docklands Consultative Committee 1990: 15).

Ward's statement also reflects, in the horrible jargon prevalent in LDDC documents during the first phase of its activities, the central significance of the doctrine of leverage – the attraction of private funding by the expenditure of public funds. Originally, the intention had been to secure a ratio of around 5:1; but in the heady days of the later 1980s this expanded to a point where claims that a much higher ratio had been achieved were freely made. These claims are suspect, to the extent that they do not reflect the substantial quantity of public funds invested either before the LDDC came into existence or subsequently through other channels; they also had to be revised downward substantially when the economic climate changed. Their significance in this context is that they provided the basic rationale for a continued high level of public sector investment – a position enthusiastically endorsed, it perhaps hardly needs stating, by the main potential beneficiaries, the developers (cf. Mobbs 1986).

The LDDC's resources are managed and its powers exercised by the Board, which is appointed by the Secretary of State for the Environment and is accordingly in the rather grandiose words of a former member (Sir Andrew Derbyshire) 'accountable to the nation, not to the local communities' (quoted in Wolmar 1989). The Board's Chair throughout its life span has been a property developer; the Vice-Chair a politician with Labour links. Members of the Board could be characterised as broadly sympathetic to the government's policy objectives. Seats were reserved for representatives from all three local authorities but have been only intermittently filled (a reflection of the reservations they have had, at least until recently). The proceedings of the Board are not subject to local government legislation and are held in private, although the planning committee meetings are now open to the public.

The Board appoints the Chief Executive and lays down the operational style. Staff numbers have been kept small; as a result, as functions have expanded there has been increasing reliance on the appointment of consultants, both to carry out executive functions and to produce a lengthy series of reports evaluating progress made and exploring some of the difficult issues arising, where expertise is lacking internally or the appearance of impartiality is required. As a result, by 1987 the budget for expenditure on consultancy exceeded that for staff. The staff themselves were split into four area teams organised on a multi-disciplinary basis under an area director, with project leaders for specific initiatives. Batley comments:

This 'matrix management' makes for relatively flat hierarchical pyramids and more personal accountability than in a typical local authority department. Speedy action is not only possible but necessary given the competition within and between area teams for LDDC funds and for private sector investments. Within the corporate plan and the approved budget, the competition is between area teams to seize opportunities, prepare budgets and submit bids. At this level, planning is reactive and the bias is to action rather than to a particular outcome.

(Batley 1989: 179)

This flavour has been carried over into all the operations of the LDDC. As already indicated, no master plan exists; nor was any attempt made initially to establish the extent of need in the Docklands area itself. Under pressure the corporation and the DoE have taken two lines. The first has been that since the overarching planning mechanisms are still in place, existing statutory plans provide the essential broad context (including, presumably, the otherwise long defunct London Docklands Strategic Plan prepared by the Docklands Joint Committee). However, the LDDC has (successfully) resisted at inquiry any attempts by the boroughs to modify this structure through new local plans. This has been done in support of the second imperative – the need to respond as rapidly and flexibly as possible to the requirements of the market. As the then Chief Executive put it: 'we will be opportunity-led so that the market place has the opportunity of influencing how and where a development takes place and what form it takes' (Brownill 1990: 53). On this basis, the LDDC is, as the DoE's representatives stressed before the House of Commons Employment Committee, a public sector development agency, which, in the words of the Under-Secretary responsible, should bring 'a single-minded approach to physical regeneration' (House of Commons Employment Committee 1988b). This function, according to him, must take priority over all others defined in the Act, including the 'very small point at the very end' about housing and social facilities.

However, the absence of a plan does not preclude setting objectives or what are described as 'performance highlights'. At various stages these have been expressed in terms of targets (which will be explored in greater detail when the specific initiatives taken by the LDDC are considered). More recently, some sectors of activity (notably transport and housing) have been the subject of more detailed reviews and planning documents have been produced. But although these documents employ the terms 'strategic' they are narrowly focused on immediate action designed to unstick jamming in the mechanisms for delivery of action on the ground. As already indicated, the Corporate Plan, which might be expected to provide some policy context, is essentially a bid to the DoE for release of resources. DoE witnesses before the House of Commons Employment Committee described the process of submission as a 'repeating cycle of corporate planning'. But the context makes it clear that this is seen as a mechanism for control over project expenditure; pressed for illustrations of the way in which the process throws up errors or lessons that could be applied in other areas, the Under-Secretary responsible found himself at a loss to respond, volunteering 'a few rough edges' (nature unspecified) as the best examples that he could offer.

In sum, the style has been responsive to the market and unhindered by any significant degree of control over policy from the government department with executive responsibility for expenditure. One commonly offered explanation rests on personalities, especially those of the first Chairman (Sir Nigel Broackes) and Chief Executive (Reg Ward). The latter was said to have 'run rings round the Department of the Environment and the LDDC

Board, so that no-one else really knew what was happening in Docklands. He loved the limelight and chose projects more for their publicity value than their suitability' (Wolmar 1989).

This style has also been critical to the development of relationships with other agencies in the public sector and in particular the boroughs. At the outset, the establishment of the LDDC was subject to review as part of the legislative procedure by a House of Lords Committee which expressed some concern about working relationships with the boroughs and the representatives of local opinion. Provision was accordingly made for the introduction of a Code of Consultation. However, this code never came into force (unlike in TPDC where at least a formal obeisance to the code is maintained – see Chapter 5, p. 87). The concessions that the LDDC were prepared to make in terms of its working procedures were too limited to be acceptable to the boroughs. Perhaps this was hardly surprising, given the contrast in attitude and working procedures between the two sides. As Batley observes:

> The LDDC has an organisation adapted to the task of rapidly facilitating private investment untrammelled by the need for wide consultation. What to the LDDC appear to be the necessary organisational conditions for identifying and building on market opportunities appear to the boroughs as reactive, secretive and exclusive practices. The London boroughs are bound by their nature as large-scale, cross-service, publicly accountable organisations to consult, to follow established procedures, to decide according to agreed policy or refer back for guidance. What for the boroughs appear to be the necessary conditions for accountability and needs-based action appear to the LDDC as bureaucratic inflexibility, hierarchy and slow decision by committee.
>
> (Batley 1989: 180)

The LDDC was having none of that, as its actions over the first phase of its existence clearly demonstrated.

LDDC IN ACTION

Following other analysts, we can divide the activities of the LDDC to date (1991) into three defined periods:

1981–5: Start-up and consolidation
1985–7: Riding the boom
1988–date: Recession and retreat to consensus

The analysis that follows reflects these changes and their impact in the different areas of the LDDC's activity.

The task of physical regeneration

It has been the sheer magnitude of the urban dereliction in the Docklands area that has provided both the opportunities and one of the main obstacles to taking full advantage of them. In retrospect, the end of commercial activity in the docks seems to have come with remarkable rapidity. In the nineteenth century, the London Docks had been the biggest and busiest in the world, both in terms of activity and size. Their consolidation under the Port of London Authority in 1909 was followed by a further period of expansion; not until after the Second World War did competition from other means of moving cargo begin to threaten profits and led the PLA to begin moving their operations downstream to Tilbury. Even at the end of the 1960s, when the first two major dock closures took place at London and St Katherine's, there were still 23,000 registered dockers in East London (Widgery 1991).

But when the decline came, it was swift. The opportunity for major new developments created by the closure of the Docks and the running down of other industrial uses that had found a home alongside them – handling and manufacture of chemicals, gas and building aggregates and sugar refining – was obvious. Michael Heseltine, who claims to have become aware of the possibilities when a minister in the Heath government of the early 1970s, comes some way down the list of the perceptive. His Conservative predecessor as Secretary of State for the Environment, Peter Walker, had already commissioned the first of many major studies, the Travers Morgan report, in 1970. This review with its coyly titled options ('East End Consolidated', 'Europa', 'Waterside', 'Fun City') found favour neither with the civil servants nor the local inhabitants. But it had one major merit. Consultation on the Travers Morgan proposals provided the catalyst for the creation of the community-based groups whose active participation has been such a striking feature of the continuing debates in Docklands (Marris 1982).

When Labour returned to power nationally and at the GLC, a new approach was adopted; a planning team was established responsible to a Docklands Joint Committee, made up of the five boroughs and the GLC and an advisory group on which local groups were represented. It was this team that produced the Docklands Strategic Plan, published in 1976, which, with the amendments made in 1978 after the DJC was expanded into the Docklands Inner City Partnership, provided the focus for activity over the next five years. Against the background of the deepest cuts in public expenditure in the entire post-war period, the planners struggled to reconcile the imperative need to attract new investment with the objective of generating employment and constructing new housing for the existing inhabitants of the Docklands boroughs, while attempting to fend off a steady flow of criticism from local groups. But the dominant problem remained the sheer extent of dereliction. An independent report, *Wasteland*, published in 1980, argued that the situation at the Tower Hamlets end of Docklands suggested 'little short of a breakdown in our land use system in both public and private sectors. While the machinery, money and incentive to reverse the decline are not forthcoming, large urban areas are becoming effectively unreclaimable' (Nabarro and Richards 1980: 119). In the following year, the LDDC took up its functions.

In fact, although the development corporation sometimes chose to behave as if it had been entrusted on declaration with a wholly derelict area, it did inherit quite a substantial amount of activity from the Docklands Joint Committee. In particular, the purchase and filling in of two major docks – London and Surrey – and the draining of the Beckton marshes, provided a basis for future activity; and the development at St Katherine's Dock (World Trade Centre) had already demonstrated the development potential of proximity to the City of London. The switch of location of large parts of the newspaper industry from Fleet Street to Wapping (instigated by Rupert Murdoch) was also already well under way (Nicholson 1989).

On the basis of this experience, the LDDC's original preference was for attracting 'foot-loose' high-tech industry and media-related activity; and much of the preliminary site preparation was undertaken with this priority in mind. Although this approach had some initial success, it was overtaken in the mid-1980s by the discovery of the potential for expansion in the deregulation of the Stock Exchange (the so-called 'Big Bang'). The rush of new investors anxious to take advantage of the opportunities this presented encountered obstacles in the City of London Corporation's reluctance to sanction further development. They turned to Docklands and the Isle of Dogs where, in close proximity to the City, they found in the Enterprise Zone a tax regime of unparalleled generosity. As the LDCC explain,

> it was capital allowance incentives as opposed to rates exemptions that became the major factor – quite the reverse of what was originally envisaged. One hundred per cent capital allowances enabled developers and investors to offset the full cost of development projects against their UK tax liabilities.
>
> (London Docklands Consultative Committee 1990: 11)

Given these conditions, one developer marketing his new scheme felt able to invite potential investors to contact FREEFONE NIL TAX.

The marketing of the Isle of Dogs as 'Wall Street on water' opens the second phase of the Docklands' activities and saw the blossoming of the LDDC's reactive planning approach, with its philosophy of going for 'growth sectors', and one in particular above all others. As the Chief Executive put it in 1986, the way is open for Docklands, rich in facilities and space to work in partnership with the City . . .the City is entering into a major phase of evolution and expansion which coincides with Docklands' ability to offer uniquely convenient and appropriate space for that expansion.

(Church 1988: 199)

This was the heroic phase of 'leverage', where public money thrust on developers, either in the form of grants or hidden subsidies on land sales, could none the less reap rewards in ratios of 9, 10, even 12 to one, to report back to gratified ministers. In such an environment, the broader objectives could be left on one side in the giddy pace of expansion; and the increasing volume of complaints from the boroughs (for example from Southwark, in their evidence to the House of Commons Employment Committee) could be safely ignored. In the process some of the earlier media and 'high tech' development of which much had once been made became surplus to the new requirements, like the Limehouse studios; and many existing river front activities – which up to that point had been preserved (with their jobs) – began to present an obstacle to the new image. Quality of design, once seen as a significant objective, also ceased to rate as a significant factor. As the former Chairman of the Planning Committee, Andrew Derbyshire, put it, 'We had to nod through some awful schemes' (Wolmar 1989). No matter: riding on the back of rapidly rising land values, the expansion, now incorporating residential accommodation for city workers as well as offices, seemed set fair to continue indefinitely.

This process reached its climax in the Canary Wharf development in the centre of the Isle of Dogs (see Map 6.1). The scheme is described by the Canadian consortium Olympia & York, the firm who took over the scheme after the withdrawal of the original developer, G. Ware Travelstead, as 'not so much a building as an entire district such as Mayfair' (House of Commons Employment Committee 1988b). It was eventually to involve the construction of twenty-six separate buildings with up to 12 million square feet of floor-space, mainly intended for offices, fully computerised and air-conditioned, with a potential total workforce of 50,000 people. This would have been complemented by 'a complete range of retailing and leisure facilities' with a four-storey skylit shopping arcade. The centrepiece of the project is the 880ft tower which was completed in July 1991 and is by far the highest building in London. The entire project is budgeted at £3–4bn and will now take until at least 1996 to complete.

In its conception and execution, Canary Wharf encapsulated the limitless ambition of the expansive stage of the Docklands programme. Its architectural form, and above all its overwhelming size, have been seized upon gleefully by critics who present it as the epitome of the overweening

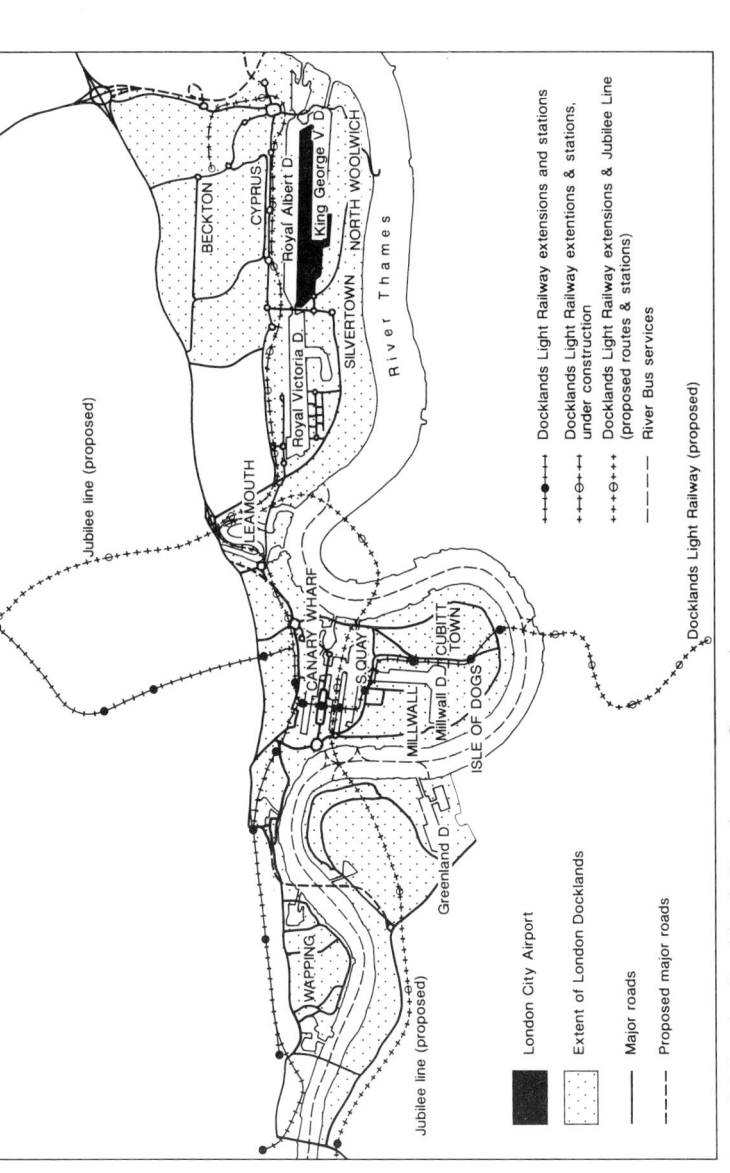

Legend:

London City Airport

Extent of London Docklands

Major roads

Proposed major roads

Docklands Light Railway extensions and stations

Docklands Light Railway extentions & stations, under construction

Docklands Light Railway extensions & Jubilee Line (proposed routes & stations)

River Bus services

Docklands Light Railway (proposed)

Map 6.1 London Docklands Development Corporation

Map labels: BECKTON, CYPRUS, Royal Albert D., King George V. D., Royal Victoria D., SILVERTOWN, NORTH WOOLWICH, River Thames, LEAMOUTH, Jubilee line (proposed), CANARY WHARF, S. QUAY, MILLWALL, Millwall D., CUBITT TOWN, ISLE OF DOGS, Greenland D., WAPPING, Jubilee line (proposed)

ambitions of the enterprise decade. 'Like Batman's Gotham city on a good day and Albert Speer's 1937 plan for Berlin on a bad one', declared the *Independent*'s architecture critic, Jonathan Glancy (*Independent*, 13 July 1991). But the debate around the scheme also contained many of the elements that helped to precipitate the subsequent change of direction and emphasis.

First, Canary Wharf posed some important questions about the terms of development. The scheme was heavily subsidised not only by application of all the Enterprise Zone concessions but also by the price at which the land was made available for the development – £400k per acre at a time when land values in and around the Enterprise Zone had risen to £3m per acre. Secondly, there were the design issues. As in the case of all developments in the UDA, the LDDC, acting as development control authority, gave planning permission without the necessity for any public inquiry. Doubts about the scale of the scheme and its impact were not confined to outsiders. Ted Hollamby, former Chief Planning Officer of LDDC (and before that Lambeth Borough Council), who resigned from LDDC in 1986, commented subsequently that 'the vast bulk and size of the buildings makes it different in scale and conception to anything in Europe, let alone London. It is not just the towers that are out of scale but the so-called "low buildings" which will completely destroy the famous view of Greenwich' (Wolmar 1989). The size and scale of the development and the numbers of workers that it will employ also had important implications for public services and in particular the capacity of the public transport system and roads to serve the new centre. Hollamby commented: 'the traffic will feed back throughout the East End. The development is proceeding so fast that everyone seems to have forgotten what the point of it is' (Wolmar 1989).

However, Olympia & York were not among the forgetful: they ensured that the Master Building Agreement would contain stipulations about the need for the development to be served by adequate public transport facilities. Equally, there were others who had not overlooked the provisions 'at the very end' of the 1980 Act and the requirement to encourage people to live and work in the area. John Mills, as Vice-Chairman of LDDC, claimed at a meeting of the Docklands Forum in 1986 that 'this many jobs coming into Docklands are bound to have an effect on local unemployment' (Church 1988: 200). A clutch of four reports on the Canary Wharf scheme produced by various consultancies came to a variety of different conclusions, the most optimistic (Henley Centre) claiming that 21,000 jobs might be gained in the three Docklands boroughs. The most pessimistic (Peat Marwick) expected that only 1,800 residents could expect to obtain employment, mostly in cleaning and catering.

These uncertainties about the likely level of benefit for local inhabitants led to attempts to secure underwriting of employment through an agreement with the developers, guaranteeing both a fixed number of jobs (2,000) for local people and a penalty in the form of a contribution to a community trust if these targets are not met. The Canadian developers, the Reichmanns, operating chiefly under North American conditions, were well accustomed to such deals being struck under the rubric of community gain and responded constructively. This raised an important question: why had LDDC made no previous attempts to secure benefits of this kind during the earlier phase of rapid expansion?

All these questions having once been aired were beginning to be debated when the period of expansion itself was brought to an abrupt halt, with the puncturing of the Stock Exchange boom (and expansion of business and jobs that went with it) after the collapse of share values across the globe on 'Black Monday' (October 1987). This event coincided with change of key personnel at the LDDC – the resignation of the first Chief Executive and departure of his successor after only two weeks in the job. Four other senior staff members and the deputy chairman also departed. Not only the style but the range and direction of the corporation's activity came under close scrutiny. The second thoughts which were the distinguishing features of the next phase of the corporation's activities towards the end of 1987 crystallised around two specific areas: jobs and housing.

Employment in Docklands

At the crest of the wave of new activity in Docklands, estimates of the numbers of new jobs that would be attracted into the area were being continually revised upwards. At the beginning of 1988, a total figure of 200,000 jobs in the area by the end of the century was being used in evidence to the House of Commons Employment Committee. However, when questioned about them, a witness from the Manpower Services Commission had the following exchange with the Committee's Chairman:

Q: These 200,000 jobs. Do you know what these jobs will be?
A: No, nor do the LDDC and nor does anyone else at the moment. You will find that estimate is a very broad brush figure and broad brush estimate and it would not be possible to desegregate it in terms of job types.

(House of Commons Employment Committee 1988b: Q 255)

Figures for past performance are rather less subject to the hazards of the broad brush, though open to a variety of interpretations. A survey was undertaken for LDDC by consultants in 1987. This found that job loss in the

Docklands area, which had continued steadily over the 1970s, had bottomed out in 1983 (when the total number of employees was 25,032) and numbers had risen thereafter quite rapidly to 42,053 at the time of the survey. Commenting subsequently on the survey, the LDDC concluded that 'Docklands, therefore, is returning to claim its historic place as a major employer and generator of growth for the London economy but this time with thriving modern growth industries which are looking towards the 21st century' (London Docklands Development Corporation 1989a).

However, the position was somewhat more complex that this statement implies. First, there is the question of the type of jobs that were being created. By far the largest growth sectors were (as would be expected) banking and finance (+495 per cent) and distribution, hotel and catering (+91 per cent). More important, the gross gain in job numbers masks losses, especially in areas which are of particular relevance for the local population. Eleven thousand jobs have been lost since declaration, mostly in manufacturing. One result of this process is that whereas 32 per cent of the total workforce lived in Docklands in 1981, this figure had declined by 1986/7 to 21 per cent. And while there is no question that new jobs had been created in Docklands, and also that there has been some benefit for locals – for example, the numbers of jobs for women have increased, though not very markedly – most of the 'new' jobs were not in fact new at all, but transfers in of staff already employed by the businesses relocating. The best that could be said, taking these additional factors into account, is that there had been a small net gain in employment over the first six years of the LDDC's life from which local people had been marginal beneficiaries. Even this much was disputed by the Docklands Consultative Committee.

In response to their criticisms, the LDDC sought first to show (following the line taken by the DoE) that employment creation was a secondary and not a primary objective for the corporation; and secondly that the loss of jobs in the traditional docklands activities that had occurred through relocation of firms had been kept to the minimum. The Acting Chief Executive claimed before the House of Commons Employment Committee that no local firms had been closed down 'of our activity' – a point strongly disputed by LDCC witnesses at subsequent hearings.

The committee itself was in no doubt about the LDDC's performance in the employment area, concluding that it is 'overtime that the corporation came to perceive that it really needed to be much more proactive in these fields' (House of Commons Employment Committee 1988a: para 39). In particular, in the area of training the corporation needed to be 'enabler, supporter and facilitator', pressing ahead with 'a broader regeneration remit' (para 44). These conclusions cannot have surprised the corporation; they echo, in terms, the scathing conclusions of the report that the LDDC had commissioned the year before from Peat Marwick McLintock. This found that the corporation's 'approach to education, training and employment has been very limited, poorly monitored and not at all successful' (para 49); and that in future 'we would expect the requirement for greater commitment from developers to employment and training initiatives to become an important feature in negotiations between the corporation and prospective developers'.

This catalogue of failures was potentially of particular significance in addressing the high rates of unemployment in the area. If the type of new economic activity that developers were bringing in provided few opportunities for local people and no special steps were taken to provide direct access to them, or for training for any other forms of employment, the prospects for reduction of unemployment in the resident population were clearly not strong. It is true that evidence for the period after 1981 shows that unemployment in the area began to fall after 1985; but this reflected national trends and the rate of reduction was not as high as in London as a whole (Brownill 1990: 99). As a result, the unemployment rate in the Docklands boroughs remained high: for instance, in 1987, the rate for Tower Hamlets was 20.8 per cent, compared with a Greater London rate of 7.5 per cent. In these circumstances, the acting Chief Executive's pledge to bring the rate *below* that for Greater London (quoted above) seems all the more surprising.

Such a pledge would only have had real meaning if attached to a far more substantial programme of job creation and training. The flaws in the first have already been set out; but the failures in the second area, at least until recently, are equally striking and attracted the ill-concealed scorn of the Chairman of the House of Commons Committee (Mr Ron Leighton) at their hearings. The sum total of the planned intervention was support for the ITEC (seventy places) – a relict of earlier attempts to attract industry based on information technology to the area – and participation in Skillnet, a joint scheme linking providers of training and mainly financed by the European Community. It took six years (a period of time repeated by the Chairman at hearings with unvarying incredulity) for the LDDC to make effective links with the Manpower Services Commission and help to establish a Docklands Liaison Group. The MSC London regional director, in his evidence, observed that 'There was the setting up of Skillnet which we joined in three years ago which was from where I saw a marked change (in LDDC attitudes)'. The exchange (with the Chairman) continued as follows:

Witness: So we were actually talking to them.
Q: You were actually talking to them. That sounds as though it is a big deal.

A: No, Sir, no. My perception of their perception was changing.

Q: In what way was it changing?

A: They were coming off what the Bishop (of Stepney) described as the glossy public relations stance and were more ready to talk to us, to local communities and the local authorities.

(House of Commons Employment Committee 1988b: A.241–3)

It would be wrong to suggest, however, that no developers who committed themselves to Docklands were interested in training issues. David Dickinson of Rosehaugh Stanhope, whose proposed scheme for the Royal Docks would have held out substantial prospects for community benefit, giving evidence in the next session, commented that 'a socially aware developer can fulfil a useful role' and singled out training as an example. But in his statement of evidence, he added:

> In my opinion, the LDDC have not been particularly successful in their early years, either in optimising the timing of cleaning out the old uses to reduce the down turn effect on local jobs or in winning the hearts and minds of the people to support their policies in seeking to create the new and potentially longer lasting jobs in the new technologies. They have certainly not been successful, to date, in obtaining the commitment of local trainers to implement long-term redirection of their training pro- grammes to produce the right skills over the next decade or more, or even made real progress in accurately identifying and promulgating the nature and numbers of these skills.
>
> (House of Commons Employment Committee 1988b: 69)

Against this background, with market-led changes still in full flow and the size and composition of the population altering rapidly in response, the risk that the existing population would be squeezed out or at best marginalised was clearly still strong. In this process, the availability of affordable housing is likely to be a factor almost as important as that of accessible and adequately-paid jobs.

Housing

The provision of housing was one of the key elements in the original local authority-led London Docklands Strategic Plan. In it, there was a strong emphasis on the provision of rented housing – half the proposed 23,000 new homes were to come from that sector and only 205 were to be owner-occupied (Nicholson 1989). The actual course of events – especially during the expansionist phase of the LDDC's activities – reversed those proportions. The development corporation, though technically not a housing authority, has had a major impact on the local housing market; having taken over a large proportion of the boroughs' land bank it leased large quantities of land to developers for construction of new housing (largely flats) for sale. Of the 15,220 new dwellings constructed in the area between designation and March 1991, 81 per cent have been built by private developers and a further 14 per cent by housing associations. Only 804 in all were built by the local authorities (London Docklands Development Corporation 1991).

The result of this activity was a dramatic shift in the tenure mix in the area from 5 per cent of dwellings in owner-occupation in 1981 to 44 per cent in 1989. Some attempt was made initially to ensure that a proportion of the new housing would be accessible to local people. A price limit of £40,000 was set, below which housing was said to be 'affordable' and priority was given to those who could demonstrate local residence. In practice, only a minority were able to take advantage of this concession; 12 per cent of those buying in this category were former Council tenants and even here there was some evidence of distortion as a result of manipulation of the rules for quick profit.

Another obstacle was that three-quarters of the new housing constructed was flats, two-thirds of them with only one or two bedrooms. The construction of large speculative high density developments near the edge of the City set off a boom in house prices, which tripled on average between 1984 and 1987, only to collapse again after Black Monday.

Caught in a declining market, developers scrabbled frantically for new customers, with price cuts and increasingly exotic inducements to buy; but this hyperactivity failed to prevent one major firm (Kentish) from going into early receivership, to be followed by a series of others as the recession deepened. Nor did it benefit local residents. The local authorities were in no position to help them. Not only had they lost most of their building land but their HIP allocations from central government had been severely cut and they were also facing the increasing costs of rehabilitating the system-built tower blocks which are the East End's characteristic public housing form. Housing associations were hardly better placed, with their allocation from the Housing Corporation showing a small decline in real terms over the period since declaration. The rapid rise in homelessness in the area between 1981 and 1988 (284 per cent increase, compared with 66 per cent in Inner London) was a clear signal of the increased pressure on affordable accommodation.

In these circumstances, the LDDC began to rethink their position. Characteristically, this took the form of commissioning reports from consultants (Coopers & Lybrand); these in turn led to the resurrection of the concept of providing 'social housing' as a policy aim and eventually to the publication of a Housing Strategy Review (1989). This envisaged the construction of

2,000 new homes, 1,200 of which would be for rent. The cost of this programme would be £70m, of which £20m would take the form of aid to the boroughs for their refurbishment programme.

This new departure for the corporation came at a time when it was also under heavy pressure to improve its performance on jobs and training. After the fundamental review of policy that had been undertaken in 1988, the corporation had held a special discussion at Board level about links between employment, education and training initiatives (Employment Policy Review, para 6.3). As a result, new priority was assigned to these areas. To provide focus for these activities, a new Community Services Directorate was created, with divisions dealing with social housing, education and training, joint programmes and child care, and the Director of the National Association of Citizens' Advice Bureaux (Elizabeth Filkin) was headhunted to fill it.

These new departures in policy formed the core of the LDDC's new approach; but one of the major questions that the Corporation had to face was resourcing them, now that the property value escalator up which LDDC and developers had ridden at a dizzy pace in the mid-1980s had turned abruptly downwards. The DoE was the only possible place to turn to; in an unpublished letter making the case for an increased allocation the Director of Finance wrote, in a brave attempt to put a favourable gloss on force of circumstances:

> The Corporation up to 1986 operated largely as a public sector development agency concentrating on physical regeneration and economic activity, the majority of expenditure being concentrated on land assembly and direct servicing of sites. By 1986, it was apparent that this strategy had been highly successful and considerable development momentum had been achieved . . . . Both the Corporation and the department perceived that reclamation of derelict land and general infrastructure improvements were not all that was required to achieve regeneration and a balanced and harmonious community.
>
> (London Docklands Consultative Committee 1990: 58)

But there were other, even more insistent, claims being pressed for additional resources which required even more urgent action and helped to precipitate a series of financial crises.

Transport

The LDDC's approach to the provision of better communications in Docklands has been based largely on new provisions which would enhance the image of the area as one in which new, high-technology solutions were adopted to provide solutions that would serve the area into the twenty-first century. The three main schemes promoted have been the Docklands Light Railway (DLR: this was in fact inherited from the London Docklands Strategic Plan), the Thamesline riverbus service and the London City Airport. But in practice, so far from providing the model for twenty-first century development, all three were by the late 1980s proving inadequate to meet the area's needs.

The DLR has been described by the LDDC as 'the cornerstone of the Corporation's commitment to increasing and improving public transport in Docklands' (London Docklands Consultative Committee 1990: 37). Phase One of the DLR links the City (Tower Gateway) with the Isle of Dogs, running down to the Southern end (Island Gardens). An extension runs northward to Stratford, where it connects with the Central Line. But, as office and residential development entered the phase of rapid expansion, it became rapidly evident that the capacity of the DLR (at 1,500 passengers per hour) would be insufficient to meet the demands of the rapidly growing population of commuters. Upgrading of the system to double-length trains and higher frequency of services from Tower Hill were accordingly introduced; but it is clear that this will be quite inadequate to meet the additional demand that will be generated by new construction, even if a reliable service can be maintained (a heroic assumption, on the basis of performance to date). In an attempt to focus effort more effectively, the decision was taken to transfer responsibility for the DLR from London Transport to the Docklands Development Corporation. This transfer took effect on 1 April 1992, on which day a points failure immobilised traffic on the Stratford branch line.

The problem with the other two high profile transport initiatives has been quite the opposite. The riverbus service is generally seen as expensive, badly integrated with other forms of transport (LRT travelcards are not accepted) and under-utilised (London Docklands Consultative Committee 1990: 40). London City Airport, launched with much fanfare, has so far proved unable to attract any significant proportion of the market in City-based commuters to Europe. After a much-disputed public inquiry, permission was secured for an extension of the runway to allow for the introduction of scheduled services by jet aircraft (previously, the use of the airport had been restricted to turbo-prop services). The first of these, to Zurich, began operating in April 1992; but the commercial viability of these services still remained in doubt.

Behind these setbacks lies a larger question: that of the absence in LDDC's earlier years of any coherent approach to communications in Docklands. Access has always been an issue; the original docks were deliberately made inaccessible to discourage piracy and pilfering. Public transport – both bus and underground – has for many years been agreed to be wholly unsatisfactory. The importance of matching provision with need was self-evident. A former Board member, Wyndham Thomas, described LDDC's approach as showing a 'woeful disregard for commonsense planning practice, such as. . .keeping infrastructure provision (especially public transport) in line with development' (London Docklands Consultative Committee 1990: 36). But 'commonsense planning practice' was precisely not what LDDC in its expansionary phase was about.

As with many other key issues in the evolution of LDDC, it was the Canary Wharf scheme that brought the contradictions to the surface. It was plainly evident to the developers that existing and planned provision for communications was entirely inadequate and would have to be supplemented – hence, the provision for upgrading in the master building agreement. But the key question was not just what should be done, but – just as with TPDC – who should pay for it. The developers' technique for dealing with this situation was simple; political pressure, applied if necessary at the top through the Prime Minister's Office (Paul Riechmann, it was said, 'enjoyed an undoubted personal chemistry with Mrs Thatcher' (*Independent*, 11 August 1991)), to secure honouring of the undertakings that facilities would be improved. Thus began what has been aptly described as a process of 'reverse leverage', by which increasing quantities of public money have been devoted to what Brownill calls 'a desperate and costly attempt to upgrade the transport infrastructure after the event' (Brownill 1990).

The most dramatic example of this process was the proposed replacement of local access roads by a new Docklands Highway, a 7.5 mile stretch of road from Beckton to Tower Hill, interlinking with the A13. At the same time, proposals were put forward for further extensions to the DLR (through the Royal Docks to Beckton) and a direct link to the main underground system at Bank station. More ambitious still, a new section of the Jubilee Line, linking Westminster and Waterloo to Canary Wharf, Greenwich and West Ham ('Canaryloo'), was proposed and the notion of a new East London river crossing, once a favoured concept among London transport planners, revived.

Initially, the government attempted to fund these ambitious new public transport initiatives by securing a substantial contribution from the developers. But developers' prospective profit margins had fallen dramatically after the collapse of the Lawson boom, and the proportion of public funding that had to be committed to secure implementation of the schemes accordingly had to be increased. When the government commissioned a consultancy report, the East London Rail Study, which strongly supported the principle of the Jubilee Line extension, a 'high-level poker game' ensued (*Economist*, 5 August 1989) as a result of which the developers' contribution to the costs of construction was further reduced to a total grant of £400m, payable in instalments. As for the road building programme, the main cost (£640m, including £220m for the mile-long Limehouse Link alone) was borne by the LDDC's own budget, together with £240m for the DLR extension.

Expenditure on this scale inevitably squeezed out alternatives, leaving the corporation to depend on receipts from land sales and deals with developers to support community projects. By September 1990, the estimated cost of the Limehouse Link had increased to £300m and, according to the Press, the Treasury was 'seeking substantial cuts and redundancies or sackings are expected'. Most of the corporation's 'social projects', which include funding playgroups and small businesses, are expected to suffer. Such cuts are likely to worsen LDDC's relations with Dockland communities (*Independent*, 16 September 1990).

Something had to give – and once again, as in 1987, 'heads rolled'. The new Chief Executive was Eric Sorensen, a DoE under-secretary and former head of their Inner Cities division. The task of the new regime was to reconcile the imperative need to fund and execute the transport and infrastructure plans as rapidly as possible with the preservation of the social programmes and in particular the task of making good the now fully-recognised deficiencies in the social housing and training programmes. On these depended the viability of the new relationships that were being made with the boroughs, which will become increasingly significant as the LDDC moves into the last phase of its life and begins to run down its activities in preparation for handing responsibility back to the boroughs. In this process, the image presented by the corporation has been a crucial element.

Image

One of the problems for LDDC in attempting to project a different image after 1987 was that it was in such sharp conflict with the one energetically cultivated at the outset. The stress on the uniqueness of the business opportunities; the 'lifestyle' advertisements (windsurfing in the docks) and hard selling of waterfront flats to prosperous young incomers and the 'clean' high-tech activities in Wapping, were all combined in one package to produce an image that excluded the existing inhabitants. So successfully was this done that some of the early incomers were astonished and disconcerted to find themselves living in close proximity to council housing estates. Equally seriously, this image was one that came to be increasingly at odds with the actual course of events, as the switch to large-scale office development followed by the downturn in property values inflicted near fatal damage on the 'twenty-first century city' concept.

More fundamentally still, after 1987 the national mood began to change; and the LDDC had always chosen to present itself as being responsive to the national interest. The setbacks in the City's fortunes – and more particularly those of the 'overpaid' young associated both with the money market and with Docklands itself – were generally greeted with ill-disguised glee. Nor could these criticisms be dismissed as the squeezings of sour grapes from opponents of the enterprise culture, locally or nationally. The developers themselves, on whose good graces LDDC depended, joined in. In his evidence to the House of Commons Employment Committee, David Dickinson of Rosehaugh Stanhope commented when questioned on relations between local people and LDDC that

> one of my strongest beliefs is that London Docklands has won only one public relations war. A lot is happening down there and they have managed to create that image. They have not won the war of suggesting that it is a nice place to be and a place that you would want to go and bring up your children, and that is because the objective they started out with was, I think, too narrow.
>
> (House of Commons Employment Committee 1988b: A 283)

The attempt to construct a new image began with a recognition that some of these comments, at least, were justified. It was reinforced by the criticisms in the House of Commons Employment Committee report and those in the corporation's own consultancy reports. It involved abandoning the style of the first Chief Executive (who 'couldn't stand talking to the locals' (Wolmar 1989)) and adopting a new, more open approach. It involved developing and publicising new policies on social housing training and child care, and wherever possible local voluntary organisations. It also involved taking a far more positive line towards collaboration with other statutory agencies – despite a warning in January 1990 from the DoE about assuming competence in areas in which the corporation had no powers (London Docklands Consultative Committee 1990: 59). And in particular, it involved a change of approach towards the once-despised boroughs.

The boroughs themselves had also rethought their position after 1987. The original line of non-collaboration was abandoned by Tower Hamlets after it passed from Labour to Alliance control in 1986, where it remained after 1990. After some hesitation, Newham followed suit. Only Southwark, by now under 'new urban left' management, maintained its intransigent position. This opening enabled the LDDC to negotiate agreements with both Newham and Tower Hamlets. Although these took a different form, in essence they rest on a similar concept: in exchange for dropping any objections that they might otherwise have made as plan-making and road authorities to the LDDC's schemes, the two boroughs will receive substantial benefits in the form of social housing and social development programmes.

At the same time, the corporation began to develop its own social programmes by commissioning further studies and engaging in systematic consultation on the form of these programmes. Although the result of the bid for resources for this purpose to the DoE was disappointing, LDDC did succeed in obtaining an allocation of £51m for such benefits in 1989/90, £8.84m of which was allocated to implementation of the two agreements and the rest divided between education, health, training (£9.98m), leisure and recreation and grants to voluntary organisations (£1.57m).

Despite these significant new departures, the likelihood that the existing resident community would achieve substantial gains from the LDDC's change of direction rested not so much on the corporation's own policies as on the possibility of extracting significant concessions from the developers who were still bringing the bulk of the new investment into the area – especially in the two major developments, Canary Wharf and the projected scheme for the Royal Docks. In short, the concept of 'community gain' to complement the financial gain that the Corporation had emphasised – to the virtual exclusion of other objectives – in the second phase.

The deal made with Olympia & York at Canary Wharf to secure more local employment was linked to the creation of a community trust. This concept was familiar to the developers as a result of their experience in North America with the 'linkage system', which requires developers to barter contributions to community needs for planning permission. Local community leaders were initially enthusiastic about the prospect of dealing direct with developers. However, in practice, performance in achievement of local jobs under the Master Building Agreement has not so far matched undertakings given, for which the downturn in property values and high interest rates is blamed. The Director of the community project created to encourage local recruitment resigned in July 1990, complaining of 'lack of cooperation, political gamesmanship and poor management' (Widgery 1991: 218). Alternative schemes are busily being devised; support for community arts and local voluntary activities, funded not only by Olympia & York but by other prominent local stakeholders, who have in some cases created their own trusts. But the Royal Docks scheme in which such hopes had been placed has collapsed and the site is now being remarketed. Developers increasingly have other issues to worry about – sheer survival, in some cases. Should community dissatisfaction with their performance persist, it is likely to be more damaging to the reconstruction of the Docklands' image than any failures on the part of LDDC itself in its own social action programmes. In particular, the dominant (in every sense) role of Canary Wharf – and the direct association of the government and senior politicians with the project – guarantees that events on the scheme will secure maximum publicity and evoke responses both locally and nationally.

So it was that the sudden financial crisis that enveloped Olympia & York as a result of the worldwide downturn in the property market in 1991 attracted attention back to the whole question of the viability of economic regeneration driven by speculative investment in commercial property. The glut in the market for office accommodation – partly as a result of the boom in construction in the City itself – drove Olympia & York to increasingly desperate measures in their attempts to let offices at Canary Wharf, including hidden or open subsidies and rent holidays. In these attempts to attract new tenants the issue of accessibility was crucial as was the chronic unreliability of the prospective tenants. In April 1992, Olympia & York, already in deep financial difficulty through heavy debts to their bankers, defaulted on the first instalment of £40m due as their contribution towards the construction of the Jubilee Line extension. Without it, plans for the extension went into abeyance. Canary Wharf itself, its offices substantially under-let and the shops serving the development mostly empty, had begun to resemble a ghost town, 1980s-style.

CONCLUSIONS

As will already be amply evident, the LDDC has had a rough ride from some of its critics, especially over the second five years of its existence. The main criticism has come from the locally-based organisations that are themselves the product of an earlier stage of public sector activity in the Docklands: the London Docklands Consultative Committee and the Docklands Forum. The GLC, having brought locally-based groups into the planning process (even if only on the margin) during the period when it was still largely responsible for the implementation process, continued to fund them, at a still higher level, from the stage when it lost those responsibilities up to the point of its own abolition. Mackintosh and Wainwright comment on this phase that

> those critics would say that concrete [sic] gains were few, the material and political impact of the GLC was considerable. By supporting local groups, the GLC was able, for a short time, to lift the low morale in Docklands and help to generate and build on existing political confidence and self organisation, most of which has outlasted the GLC itself.
>
> (Mackintosh and Wainwright 1987: 300)

The Consultative Committee's analyses of progress have been based throughout on a consistent position: rejection of the notion that local authorities have only a marginal role to play in regeneration and on an affirmation of the right of local people to closer involvement in the process of redevelopment. While some of those concerned were at the time among the strongest critics of the Docklands Joint Committee's proposals, they now retrospectively identify the needs-based planning approach of the DJC with its emphasis on public-sector-led solutions to problems of housing and employment as an altogether more satisfactory alternative. It would be fair to add that the LDCC has close links with Labour-controlled local authorities in London, so their position on these issues is perhaps not an entirely surprising one.

The Docklands Forum – which was funded first by the GLC and then after its demise in part by the London Boroughs Grants Committee – has provided a vehicle for the expression of some of the general objections to the market-led approach of the LDDC, with its heavy emphasis on physical development. Some of the members of the forum are lobbying groups formed during the 1970s in the earlier phase of Docklands planning; others are church-based or represent specific interests (Tower Hamlets Association for Racial Equality); still others are local residents' groups. (There is some suggestion that there is little community of interest between these different categories of group.) From being part of the planning process in the 1970s, when the Forum had a seat on the DJC, it has found itself, at least until 1987, very much on the outside. As its Chair commented in his evidence to the House of Commons Employment Committee:

> The difficulty to date has been the complete absence of any formal structure which we could use with the local authorities or which would work directly with the community organisations. This is in the sense of getting access to a point where decisions are made and being able to make an input into them and being able to achieve changes.
>
> (House of Commons Employment Committee 1988b: A 628)

The Forum and LDCC have therefore spoken as outsiders, perhaps understandably resentful at their complete exclusion until recently from the planning process. But one clear merit of their position and the way in which it has been argued is that an alternative agenda has been on offer from the very beginning of the Docklands experience – and was argued in the House of Lords before LDDC was declared. The problem has been that it could be dismissed (as it was by the House of Lords) as essentially a parochial position, inappropriate to the conduct of business in a development of such obvious national policy significance.

As we have seen, the LDDC's dismissive view of the position articulated by the LDCC and the protests of local groups (not the same thing) has been somewhat modified recently. At the same time, local attitudes have also changed. Although the LDDC may not be around for very much longer, the physical evidence of their activity is plain to see and will not disappear with the corporation. As the Chair of Docklands Forum put it, 'if space in Canary Wharf is built and then filled' and if 'developments in the Royal Docks go ahead, then that will create something large scale that is very permanent. It is not fly-by-night any more' (House of Commons Employment Committee 1988b: A 626).

In some respects, the changes that will be brought about if the LDDC's transport programme is carried to a successful conclusion will be even more dramatic: the geographical isolation of the traditional East End will finally be broken down and connections will be opened up not just to the City and West End, but southwards across the river and to the east along the Thames.

Something of the same feeling that irreversible changes were taking place seems to have been behind the change of attitude in two of the three boroughs, as the time approaches when they will have to take on responsibility for whatever LDDC leaves behind. The agreements reached with Tower Hamlets and Newham represent an attempt from both sides to bridge the gap; but the knock-on effects of the miscalculations and errors of judgement on the transport programme have put the financial support for these programmes in jeopardy. If this is not rapidly put right, failure to deliver the promised benefit may well sour relations again and add to the awkwardness of the final transitional stage.

Alongside the changes in the physical environment, other changes in the size and composition of the population that have taken place are almost equally certain to last. In the Isle of Dogs, the two communities – the existing East-enders and the incomers – will have to learn to live with one another. If David Widgery is right, the main obstacles that will have to be surmounted are not so much contrasting lifestyles as differences in life chances. The vast and visible disparities in wealth and housing circumstances that are every visitor's abiding impression of the 'New' East End will not readily disappear, even if the LDDC's social programmes eventually acquire and sustain a modicum of the momentum of their earlier physical regeneration initiatives.

Having said this, most observers are prepared to take the LDDC's change of direction as genuine; but many of them (not just the LDCC) have doubts about their capacity to fund and sustain them in the changed economic environment of a substantial recession, affecting both public and private sectors. The glut of office accommodation means that the alternative funding option of selling land for development is unlikely to raise new funds on a scale sufficient to underpin a major programme. Over the longer term, the pattern is turning out to be the opposite of that envisaged by the first Chief Executive – not 'frontloaded' but backweighted.

The joker in the pack is the DoE: if the department is prepared to allow expenditure on social programmes to take higher priority and fund them at a level that prevents them from being crowded out by pressing infra-structure items, then there may be some prospect that the LDDC will hand over to the boroughs an area that is socially as well as economically viable, in terms of the 'very small point at the very end' of Section 136 of the Act. With their own man in the post of Chief Executive and the admonitions of the National Audit Office on keeping a stronger grip on priorities clearly on record (National Audit Office 1988) that becomes a feasible option. The renewed concern at national level about promotion of good-quality training has obvious relevance for policy priorities in Docklands. But if public-sector-led *dirigisme* is brought into play in this way, what then becomes of the claim that Docklands incarnates market-based solutions to inner city regeneration?

Certainly, events up to 1987 offer no evidence that a market-led approach will move into equilibrium of its own accord – still less that public funding can be tapered off even if development moves ahead again. In this sense, the Treasury can be seen to have been entirely right (in their own terms) in their opposition to Heseltine's original plans for UDCs as offering 'a wide opening for additional public expenditure' (Heseltine 1987). That is exactly what it has turned out to be – £1.3bn in direct subsidy so far and more, not less, every year. And this discounts the hidden subsidy of the Enterprise Zone tax allowances, up to 1992, which have been calculated at £1.3bn (London Docklands Development Corporation 1991) and other public spending in the area. The attempt to cream off development profits for transport infrastructure having ended in fiasco, total public expenditure under that head up to 1995 is now estimated at £2.3bn. If, as Heseltine also observed in his book (p. 147), 'the Treasury never sleeps', this whole episode must have been a waking nightmare for them.

A provisional balance sheet

This is more difficult to strike than the profusion of documentation might suggest. The claims made on the corporation's behalf are encapsulated in Michael Heseltine's Tenth Anniversary speech: Docklands has been a 'tremendous success', which is reflected in £8.4bn of private investment; 27m square feet of new commercial floorspace; 600 hectares of reclaimed land; £3.5bn worth of new roads and railways; 5,000 new homes, 200 from housing associations; 1,300 improved council houses; 41,000 jobs and £20m of training and education grants (London Docklands Development Corporation 1991). But although the figures have a fine ring, none of this is conclusive. If set in the context of targets, it might be more impressive: but such targets as were from time to time set are clearly still far out of reach: 200,000 jobs (kindly characterised as 'broad brush') are unattainable in present circumstances: 30,000 dwellings, referred to in 1989 as the aspiration for 1995, await the recovery of the London housing market. For the present, new private housing construction in Docklands has ceased altogether.

The fabled leverage ratio might offer a more objective form of test: the difficulty here is the basis on which it is to be calculated. If only the DoE base grant is categorised as public expenditure, then on the LDDC figures used by the Secretary of State a ratio of 6.3:1 can be claimed – not the spectacular level of the middle eighties, but well within the range originally being aimed at. But if the additional expenditure on transport infrastructure is included (which, since the Secretary of State included it in his list of achievements, seems legitimate) and the Enterprise Zone concessions are added, then the ratio sinks to 3.4:1 – hardly the kind of standard under which flagships can sail in triumph.

The critics, of course, employ quite other criteria. They would wish, first of all, to refer to the total pattern of expenditure – how the cake was cut, in the time-worn image (see Table 6.2).

Their other tests include the extent to which locals have obtained access to new jobs, continuing rates of unemployment, the construction or re-furbishment of homes for locals and the level of homelessness. On most of these criteria, the performance of the LDDC has been indifferent (see Table 6.3). Of the 41,000 jobs referred to by the Secretary of State, 24,500 are transfers with incoming employers – less than 17,000 are genuinely new. Taken together with job losses over the same period of 20,000 the net balance over the decade is a minus quantity (3,670, to be precise). Lack of access for locals to such new employment as has been created is reflected in the persistent high rates of unemployment in the Docklands wards. In April 1991 the Department of Employment's figures showed a rate of 17.2 per cent in these wards, two-and-a-half times the Greater London average. Furthermore, these figures have been rising steadily since the beginning of 1990. Although substantial investment has recently gone into education and training, the LDDC still only supports 5,000 places in the entire Docklands area.

On housing, the LDDC's Social Housing Strategy set a target of 2,000 new build units; but cuts in the 1991 budget make it almost certain that this target will not be reached (see Table 6.4). Refurbishment of local authority housing units is projected to increase; but a substantial sum will have to be diverted from the programme to rehouse households made homeless by the building of the Limehouse Link road.

Could it have been done better if a different approach had been adopted?

Table 6.2 LDDC income and expenditure, 1981–90

	£m	%
Income		
Grant-in-aid	1,100	79.0
Sales of land and property	275	19.7
Other	18	1.3
Total	1,393	100.0
Expenditure		
Staff salaries/administration	136	10.2
Environment	72	5.4
Land acquisition	155	11.6
Land reclamation	113	8.5
Utilities	142	10.6
Roads	344	25.8
Industry/community support	65	4.9
Housing	147	11.0
DL Railway	158	11.8
Publicity	3	0.2
Total	1,335	100.0

Source: Hansard, 2 May 1991

'It is easy to forget. . .how Docklands might look today without the LDDC', says Michael Heseltine. This is the General Wade syndrome, after the Hanoverian General who pacified the Highlands – 'If you'd seen all those roads before they were made/You'd lift up your hands and bless General Wade'. The point is that we can't bless General Wade, or praise the LDDC by reference to the past, merely for saving us from an unknown alternative, because there is no knowing what would have happened if they hadn't done things in their chosen way. It's possible to hypothesise that a Docklands

Table 6.3 Employment in Docklands, 1981–90

Total Jobs Attracted	41,421
Transfers	24,559
New Jobs	16,862
Total Jobs Lost	20,532
Net Loss	3,670

Source: Hansard, 8 May 1991

Table 6.4 Social housing expenditure in Docklands, 1981–90

	1981/2	1982/3	1983/4	1984/5	1985/6	1986/7	1987/8	1988/9	1989/90	1990/1
New Units (£m)	0	0	3.3	0	0	0	0	50.5	43.7	27.0
Refurbishment (£m)	0	0.4	0.4	0	0.2	1.7	2.3	6.8	2.8	8.5

Source: Hansard, 8 May 1991

Joint Committee properly funded by a Labour government re-elected in the 1978 General Election that in real life James Callaghan fatally declined to hold, might have broken the log-jam and produced a revitalised East London with a different mix of jobs and housing. Much depends on your assumptions and on the power of your imagination. The ready dismissal of the record of the LDDC's predecessors has become part of the stock-in-trade of the LDDC's apologists – and even of some of their critics. Nicholas Faith concludes his jeremiad:

> Whatever problems the Reichmanns may face, whatever you think about the architecture of Canary Wharf, or the gigantic sums of public money now being spent on Docklands, Londoners can only blame themselves for not taking the opportunity earlier, more coherently, and more imaginatively.
>
> (*The Independent*, 11 August 1991)

We were all guilty, it seems.

Meanwhile, in the real world, the rival claims for disaster and triumph all seemed until recently somewhat exaggerated, at least, until the spectacular collapse of Olympia & York into receivership, under the impact of the worldwide property recession. The collapse (which occurred after this book went to press) compromised any immediate prospect of funding the extension to the Jubilee line and remedying the crucial weakness of the whole Docklands scheme: inadequate communications. It also provoked a renewed crisis of confidence in the future viability of the Docklands as an exercise in urban renewal, which was still far from being resolved at the time of writing (September 1992). Even so, Docklands has neither demonstrated the unquestionable superiority of market-led regeneration and led to the 'death of planning' nor demonstrated the hollowness of claims for the enterprise culture. The physical environment has been altered out of all recognition in a remarkably short period; the quality of much (but not all) this redevelopment is – charitably – not high; but some jobs have been created as a result and the housing mix has been changed in a way which would not have seemed conceivable twenty years ago. There is, of course, a downside to these achievements, best expressed in terms of who has benefited from this process. 'Trickle down', to the extent that it has happened at all, has been selective: women have benefited, but only from the usual low-wage part-time work. There is an obvious risk of social polarisation taking place – and relying on incoming firms to display their social conscience by hiring local labour may not be sufficient insurance, especially in mid recession.

Finally, are the Docklands really a special case? Clearly from the critics' angle there is an understandable desire to show that the whole 'project' (sic) has failed and that the new right agenda associated with it can therefore be dismissed. Most other UDCs now seem to want to distance themselves from the Docklands experience; Heartlands UDA is one that does. Certainly, there is one sense in which LDDC is very much a special case. The DoE, as the department with lead responsibility for the inner cities programme, has treated it as such, both in the share of total resources that it has and in the extraordinary indulgence with which the relationship has been conducted (the National Audit Office were surely quite right to get tough about this). This indulgence reached its peak with the pouring of public money down the open drain of the Isle of Dogs Enterprise Zone. The fiasco of Olympia & York's failure to contribute to the costs of improving the transport infrastructure finally brought the curtain down on this epoch.

However, in other ways the case for Docklands' uniqueness is not strong. The area is not as large, in terms of size or population, as is sometimes implied; and the problems experienced there are in no sense worse than those on Merseyside, where a UDC was declared at the same time. It is hard to resist the notion that there's a 'London factor' at work here – the tangled past history and vendettas associated with it, but above all the sheer visibility of it all from Whitehall and Westminster. Hence the sense that this scheme simply couldn't be allowed to fail, at least as long as Margaret Thatcher and Nicholas Ridley were at their respective posts.

The final question to answer is the one with which we began: what, precisely, has been the nature of the approach being tested in Docklands? Was it in practice just another form of corporatism – or, to put it fancifully, was the flagship sailing under false colours? Near the beginning, whatever Michael Heseltine may assert in retrospect, a feeling seems to have developed that the market really could take care of it all, especially after 1983 when it looked as if the Lawson–Howe economic policies had worked. For a while, Broakes and Ward did try to run LDDC as a single-purpose physical redevelopment agency responding solely to market forces. But they became intoxicated by their success in marketing the enterprise to the City and realised too late that they were in a hole from which only more public money could float them out. Then planning returned by the back door and the failures of the *laissez-faire* era had to be put right. The incompatibility of the competing objectives that emerged as a result led in turn to a second internal convulsion and the compromise that is now in place.

This interpretation does at least have the merit of being consistent with Michael Heseltine's doctrine of responsible partnership between public and private sectors. With the benefit of John Patten's '20:20 hindsight' it is clear that the single-purpose development agency with an agenda purely determined by the market could never have produced lasting solutions that satisfied the needs of all parties – whatever his own rhetoric might have suggested. But it has little to say about the ways in which an effective social programme can be introduced and sustained. For that we must turn elsewhere.

7 Heartlands – a different approach to partnership

THE BIRTH OF THE HEARTLANDS

To the Conservative government, considering the location of new initiatives to make up the next phase of inner city policy that had opened in 1986, it must have been clear immediately that Birmingham had to be included. The city had experienced all the earlier forms of special programme, including community development projects, inner area studies, partnership committees and now city action teams. Unlike some other major cities – notoriously, Liverpool – these earlier initiatives had mostly taken root and delivered some useful outcomes. Various explanations have been offered for this; the relative lack of adversarial heat in local politics, even after the rift between local and central government had opened in the early 1980s; or the long-established willingness of the city authorities to work in close collaboration with local industry under administrations of all political colours, stretching back to the last century and Joseph Chamberlain's version of municipal socialism. But perhaps most basic of all, Birmingham had to be included because no credible inner cities programme of action could conceivably have omitted the city which would be the test case of an employment-led regeneration policy.

The effects of the deep recession of the early 1980s were particularly strongly felt in the West Midlands; the region fell precipitately from prosperity to slump as its excessive reliance on traditional manufacturing industry exposed it to the full effects of the rapid rise in unemployment brought about by national economic policies. But over and above the impact of these policies, the region was feeling the effects of fundamental structural changes in the local economy. As Spencer and his colleagues, writing in 1986, put it:

> The scale of industrial dereliction and the wholesale closure of industrial plants bear witness to the depth of the crisis which the West Midlands's industry is experiencing. . . . The landscape of the West Midlands has

been fundamentally altered. An upturn in the national economy would not by itself solve the problems of the local economy or lead to a massive reduction in unemployment in the West Midlands. The industrial capacity no longer exists there.

(Spencer *et al.* 1986)

Nowhere were the consequences of these developments more sharply felt than among the city's ethnic minority population. The sudden outbreak of violence in Handsworth in September 1985 underlined the nature and extent of the problem: though the proximate cause of the episode remained in dispute even after two rival committees of inquiry had reported (West Midlands County Council 1986), the problems faced by young blacks in a shrinking labour market with little place for unskilled and semi-skilled manual labour were beyond dispute. Concern to address these problems was reflected not only in the substantial package of new programmes assembled by the City (Birmingham City Council Handsworth Coordinating Committee: Second Report, 1988) but in the selection of the area for inclusion in the first group of Task Forces created by Kenneth Clarke in February 1986 – for whom the promotion of inner city black businesses was a key objective.

The city had also been one of the original Inner City Partnership Authorities under Peter Shore's 1977 urban policy. An evaluation of the total impact of the Partnership conducted in 1985 had reached the conclusion that the Partnership had 'helped to stabilise conditions in the inner city, despite a background of economic decline' (Aston University 1985). The city had also been assigned in 1985 one of the City Action Teams (CATs) of locally-based civil service agencies, under the leadership of the Regional Director of the DTI. By 1987, the Partnership had an overall budget of £29m, with an increasing emphasis on economic projects within the total pattern of expenditure (see Table 7.1).

Table 7.1 Birmingham inner city partnership expenditure, 1987–8

Topic	*Share (%)*	*Allocation*
Economy	35	£9.52m
Social and community	12	£3.04m
Health and PSS	9	£2.83m
Movement	8	£2.17m
Housing	10	£2.77m
Environment	15	£5.08m
Voluntary bodies	11	£3.80m
Total	100	£29.21m

A number of additional mechanisms therefore existed both for channelling further resources into high priority schemes in inner Birmingham and co-ordinating the contribution of the various agencies. Their existence also added to the number of agencies and individual actors with a stake in future developments in Birmingham's inner city areas.

By 1987 the city was beginning to make its way back towards economic equilibrium. This was partly as a result of the general recovery of the national economy in the second half of the 1980s and partly as a result of a vigorous programme of economic development spearheaded by the city and (before its abolition) the West Midlands County Council, which succeeded in attracting substantial sums from the European Commission for regeneration of the city centre. But this recovery was uneven and left large tracts of the inner city still in deep recession. This was reflected in the persistent very high rates of unemployment in inner city wards, which form a ring immediately surrounding the city centre, running clockwise from the west round to the south east.

The policy emphasis on municipally-led economic regeneration in close collaboration with the private sector was consistent with past practice in Birmingham – as, for example, in the development of the National Exhibition Centre (NEC) in the early 1970s and subsequently the construction of the International Convention Centre (ICC), which was based directly on experience with the NEC. The persistence of this climate of cooperation sets Birmingham apart from other English major cities, in particular because it is politically bipartisan. Differences over means had been quite sharp in the early 1980s, especially during the West Midlands County Council's brief span of life; but the ends – a wide spread of new jobs, with priority wherever possible for locals and broadening the economic base to reduce excessive reliance on the traditional manufacturing sector – were generally accepted. Most important in this context, the promotion of collaboration between public and private sector as the most effective way in which to deliver on these objectives was accepted by all political parties. Nor was there evidence of resistance on the part of private industry: on the contrary, the Birmingham Chamber of Commerce and Industry – one of the strongest in the country – has been a convinced advocate of such collaboration.

Thus Labour – led by Dick Knowles – coming back into office in 1984 after a brief interlude of Conservative rule, not only placed a new emphasis on the importance of economic regeneration through enhanced powers for the Economic Development Committee, whose Chairman Albert Bore was a key figure in Knowles's administration, but initiated a new series of quarterly meetings with leading figures in the local private sector. The bridge built in this way was crucial for later developments, when it had to bear the stress of a great deal of heavy traffic.

So Birmingham, Labour-controlled though it was, could not easily be categorised as being one of the 'unacceptable' local authorities with whom Conservative ministers (like Kenneth Clarke) professed themselves unable to do business. Yet to a government committed to a new departure whose main thesis was that, in John Patten's phrase, 'the public-sector dominated solutions of the past simply have not worked' (*Guardian*, 17 April 1987) and anxious above all to demonstrate that early and vigorous action was being taken, the case for including Birmingham in the next wave (Phase Three) of the UDC programme whose extension became a key 1987 Election manifesto pledge was self-evidently strong. The problem from the city's point of view was to be able to advance a sufficiently convincing alternative with a wide enough span of local support.

Immediately after the Conservatives' 1987 election victory and the Prime Minister's immediate pledge to do something about 'those inner cities', Dick Knowles as Leader of Birmingham wrote to the Secretary of State for the Environment – Nicholas Ridley – to propose a meeting and also to Lord Young, who had been transferred to the Department of Trade and Industry. Before the election, in tentative approaches to Ridley, the city had floated the notion of a joint public–private sector agency with central government core funding on the same basis, if not entirely to the same extent, as a UDC. Knowles now resumed the contact, arguing that the scale of Birmingham's problems made it essential that there should be active involvement by the public sector locally. His approach set in train a series of meetings at which the government's intentions for the city were reviewed and the case for an alternative was deployed.

To be at all convincing, the case the city was now advancing needed to be based on explicit arguments which demonstrated sound preparation and solid support from the private sector. This had become possible as the result of a series of developments that had taken place under the umbrella of the joint city–private sector consultative group set up in 1984 and with the energetic encouragement of the regional directors of the DTI and DoE. The germ of the idea had originally been advanced two years earlier by John Douglas, Managing Director of a large locally-based firm of developers, R. M. Douglas. He had developed the notion – taken from American experience – of issuing tax-exempt bonds to provide capital for extensive redevelopment in inner Birmingham. He tried this idea out on the then Regional Director of the DoE, who in turn thought it worth floating with the Treasury. Their response was (predictably, perhaps) to sink it without further ado. However, the response from both those fellow-developers whom Douglas consulted (who later made up the core of the private sector side in the negotiations) and the regional directors (who collectively made up the CAT) was sufficiently enthusiastic to justify putting a modified version into the liaison meetings with the city and thence into the wider policy arena.

Two other factors helped to add credibility. Firstly, the role of Birmingham's Chamber of Commerce both as co-ordinators and as advocates to a group of ministers still disposed to automatic hostility to proposals emanating from the direction of a local authority. The Chamber (which has over 4,000 members) has been a significant player in a number of urban regeneration initiatives, from the promotion of the NEC onwards. It has helped to promote enterprise agencies and, in collaboration with the City Action Team, it has taken a special interest in supporting Asian businesses in the city.

A second and crucial element was the existence of a plausible location for a collaborative initiative and a clear indication of what could be achieved on the selected site. The area in question was the Aston and Nechells district immediately to the east of the city centre off the inner ring motorway and close to M6 and 'Spaghetti Junction'. The area contained approximately 700 acres of vacant land; some of the industrial sites were derelict and contaminated, displaying the visible scars of the recession in the form of closed factory buildings. Much of the land was owned in small parcels, but among the existing firms were a number of substantial operators: Metro Cammell, Jaguar, DAF/Freight/Rover. The two wards also exhibited signs of acute social deprivation – Nechells was among the 10 per cent most deprived wards in England and Wales at the 1981 Census. But equally there were obvious signs of potential – a functioning canal system as well as direct access to motorway network, the neighbouring Aston Science Park, a major site (the gasworks) becoming available and the prospect of another (Fort Dunlop) providing the opportunity for high prestige developments.

In the climate of gradual economic recovery the potential for regeneration in the area seemed clear; and an initiative based on it would be wholly consistent with the economic development policies adopted after 1984. The city's approval in principle to the proposal arrived within two weeks of receiving it; and a feasibility study was then commissioned from the consultants Roger Tym, speculatively funded by the developers who had now come together in an informal consortium, with support from the City Council and the DoE. City logistic support was provided to the study by officer working parties. The location of the new initiative fitted well into the CAT's notion of a balanced approach to the problems of inner Birmingham and the Inner City Partnership's concern that too much attention and resources were being directed into Handsworth (which might be seen as 'rewarding rioting'). The useful coincidence of well-placed Ministers (like Norman Fowler) with seats in the Birmingham region, who were carefully played into the picture by the city, was also fully exploited.

By the end of 1986 the broad outlines of an alternative approach were already in place, but a necessary condition for further progress – especially in the light of the commitments subsequently entered into at the time of the election campaign – was a positive response from central government. The advocates of the alternative had a difficult hand to play and the stakes were high: the government did not hesitate to impose UDCs in Phase Three on reluctant Manchester and recalcitrant Sheffield.

But the time bought had been used to good effect. A further meeting, with Harold Musgrove from the Chamber of Commerce as leader of the Birmingham deputation, appeared to have half-convinced the Secretary of State that the alternative to the UDC now formally on offer was viable. Nevertheless, his relations with the city did not develop smoothly. On a trip to Birmingham, Ridley roundly accused the city of dragging its feet, claiming that nine months had now been wasted and that this was justification enough for taking responsibility away from the Council (*Daily News,* 2 July 1987). Albert Bore retorted that work was already far more advanced than in other areas (in particular, the Black Country) in which the government had recently established Second Phase UDCs.

Despite this discouraging public posture by the minister, the collaborators persisted and proposals in final form were presented to the Secretary of State in November 1987. The proclaimed intention was to prove that 'a local authority can collaborate with industry to revive the inner city without the imposition of a Whitehall solution'; and the minority Conservatives committed themselves to the proposal without reservation, the Chamber of Commerce commenting that 'there is a tradition of sinking political differences and working together for the good of the city'. Sweetness balanced by Dick Knowles's sour aside that the government 'don't trust local government; they don't want it to be successful' (*Guardian,* 20 October 1987).

Crux issues for final resolution were the extent to which core funding would be provided by the government; visible evidence that the private sector would take a lead, in both composition and chairing of the Board, and a commitment by the city to provide support (not just logistics but a planning regime) that approximated to that conferred on UDCs by statute. On all of these, Ridley's terms were harsh: there would be no core funding; and the original notion of a 51:49 split between public and private sector would have to be abandoned. Any notion of a joint collaboration between equal partners would have to give way to the city in a supporting and facilitating role. With little room for manoeuvre left, the bullet was bitten and an urban development authority duly constituted as Birmingham Heartlands Ltd, with 65 per cent of the shares going to the five 'founder developers' (Bryants, Douglas, Gallifords, Tarmac and Wimpey), 35 per cent to the City Council and a single share to the Chamber of Commerce, who also nominated the Chairman, the former Conservative Minister Sir Reginald Eyre. The Chief Executive was to be nominated by the developers and the Finance Director by the city. With these concessions the way was clear to proceed.

PLANNING FOR HEARTLANDS

The report produced by Roger Tym and partners had, as already indicated, played a crucial part in the politics of the establishment of Heartlands. But the consultants' report was equally significant in determining the main priorities for action in the area once the Secretary of State had given his consent.

Brisk and to the point in the pared-down variant of consultants' language, the Tym report sets out the state of the area and the impact upon it of the recession of the first half of the 1980s. A resident population of 16,656 (at the 1981 Census), with unemployment at 31 per cent in the month in which the report was presented (November 1987) reflecting the loss of a third of the jobs in the area over that period. Metal manufacturing and vehicle manufacture accounted for more than a third of the remaining jobs; negligible investment had taken place in existing small firms in the area, which contained almost 500 in 1981 partly because of a poor environment further blighted by 'bad neighbour' industry and access problems.

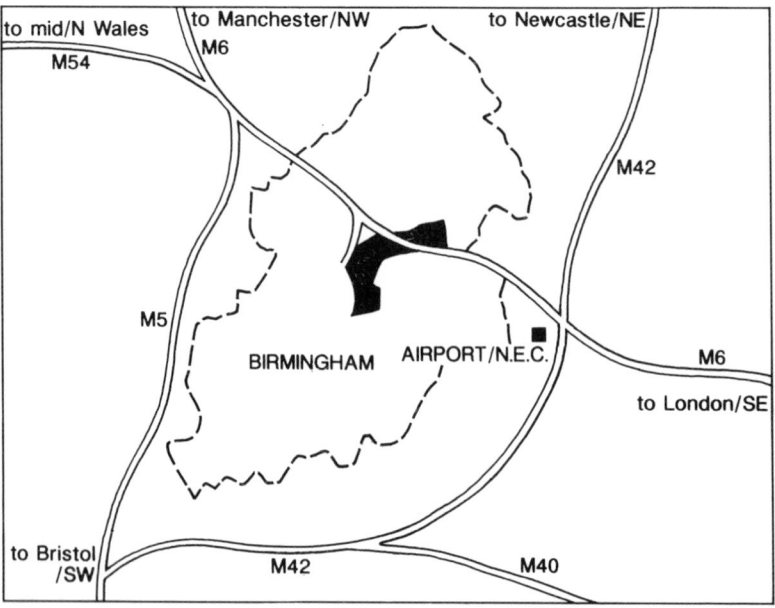

Map 7.1   Heartlands location

The social circumstances were also poor. The area contained just over 6,000 households in 1981, 81 per cent of them in council accommodation, often of low standard and only 10 per cent owner occupiers. Four out of five households neither owned nor had access to a car. There are limited educational opportunities and consequent shortage of skills in the area's resident population. Three-quarters of the heads of household at the 1981 Census were UK–born; 8.4 per cent came from the Republic of Ireland and 18.3 per cent from the New Commonwealth and Pakistan.

At the same time, the report identifies a series of opportunities: large areas of land providing early development potential; excellent accessibility once outside the cramped road system of the area itself, including access to the airport; a substantial resident work-force with potential for retraining; proximity to the Aston Science Park and the city centre; a canal system with strong potential for enhancement on which the Inner City Partnership had already spent substantial sums. And, less tangibly but politically crucial, the consultants preferred Birmingham City Council's track record of past helpfulness towards new commercial developments. Provided that a series of intermediate problems could be satisfactorily addressed – the dispersed pattern of land ownership, the confused and obsolete road network and the poor image of the area – the consultants' conclusion was that despite the competition within and outside the region (including the new Black Country Development Corporation) the potential for profitable offices, retail and some factory development was substantial. Always providing that a coherent plan to upgrade the area as a whole, linked to radical improvement in the infrastructure, was adopted and marketed.

The form that such a plan would take was sketched in: two main focuses for development, one around the canal system (rechristened 'Waterlinks'), the other at the former gasworks ('Starsite'). A new link road was needed through the centre of the area for communication purposes together with some new housing. As the consultants punctiliously observe, 'transformation of the image of the area and the attraction of new investment and residents to it should not be at the expense of existing residents' (Tym 1987a: 29). Substantial upgrading of existing local authority housing would accordingly be necessary, after an audit of community views; and a new development with mixed tenures was proposed at the Bordesley Village site. (See Map 7.2.) In undertaking these developments, care should be taken to secure responses from a full spectrum of local opinion – tenants and local employers, as well as the agencies operating locally. Funds for the whole process would need to be assembled over time from a variety of sources; on the management of the complex series of actions required by the Plan the authors are completely silent (Tym 1987a).

The Tym report set out the basic problems clearly enough for the new

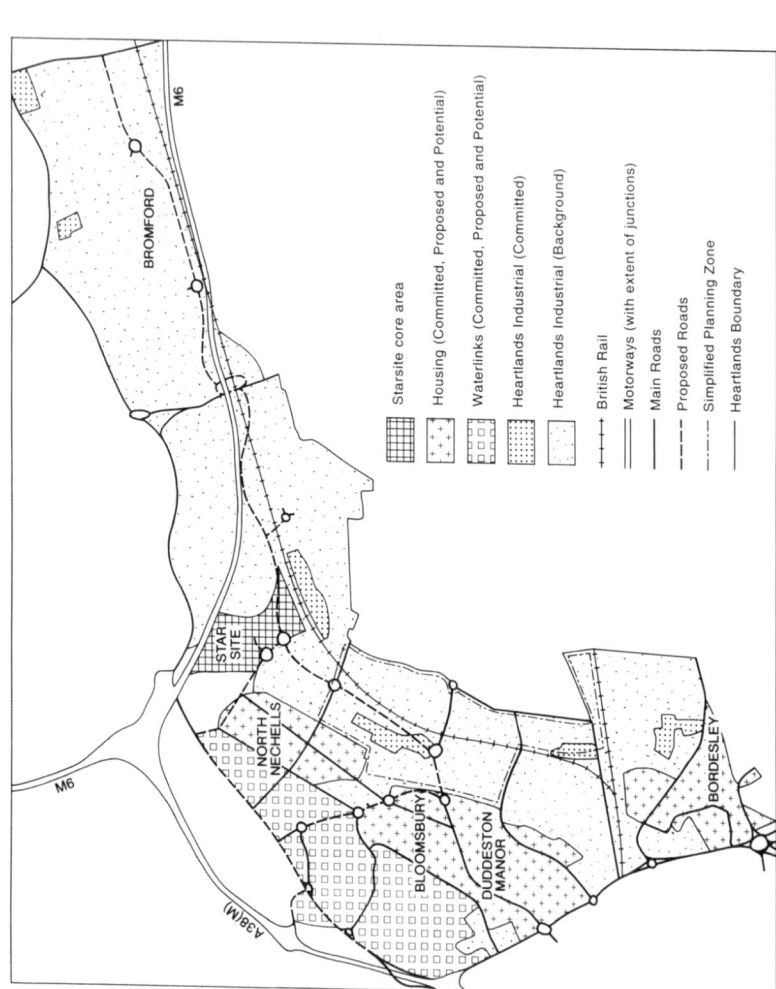

Key:

Starsite core area

Housing (Committed, Proposed and Potential)

Waterlinks (Committed, Proposed and Potential)

Heartlands Industrial (Committed)

Heartlands Industrial (Background)

British Rail

Motorways (with extent of junctions)

Main Roads

Proposed Roads

Simplified Planning Zone

Heartlands Boundary

BROMFORD

M6

STAR SITE

NORTH NECHELLS

BLOOMSBURY

DUDDESTON MANOR

BORDESLEY

A38(M)

M6

Map 7.2 Heartlands: development proposals

Heartlands Board to identify the main issues that it would have to address in the first phase of its work. As a coalition of common but distinct interests it would also be important to secure the lines of consultation both with parent agencies (notably the city's executive departments) and other active players on the local scene, in particular the Inner City Partnership with its substantial resources. As the report had stressed, local consultation would also be an important priority.

Such consultation, based on the proposals in the Roger Tym report, duly followed, with a series of exhibitions and meetings on the basis of a summary version of the report (with some minor modifications) and the addition of a proposal for a community trust to fund small-scale local schemes in the community. The consultation was launched in March 1988 with a fanfare of media publicity and provoked in response some anxieties and animosities: concern that Heartlands would go down the same track as Docklands provided the basis for demonstrations and the preparation of an alternative 'residents' plan' contrasting not only in terms of cost (£800 compared with £70k for Tym's) but in objectives, with more housing and open space and a stress on public transport.

Although opposition was not sustained and the plan was adopted by the local authority in July 1988 with only minor modifications, the consultation sent a clear warning signal. Remoteness had to be avoided; above all, the widespread local perceptions of London Docklands were not (as the government wished to present it) of successful regeneration through private enterprise but of an autocratic and unaccountable organisation responding not to local needs but to imperatives of profit maximisation and interests of new residents with no local roots – the dreaded yuppies. The Heartlands team moved itself into the area with some fences to mend.

One of the issues that had emerged clearly in the course of the consultation was the artificiality of the area designated as Heartlands, as least as far the resident population was concerned. For them there were at least four neighbourhoods, not one: Bordesley in the south, cut off from the rest by the road and rail pattern; Duddeston and Bloomsbury in the centre and, beyond a belt of industrial activity, North Nechells. The social strategy, in order to command consent (let alone community participation), would have to reflect the existence of these separate entities – and also the lack of adequate social facilities within these areas. At the same time, the industrial strategy would have to confront a different sort of heterogeneity – the variety of uses and 'checkerboard' of land ownership with some owners markedly reluctant to surrender control (see Map 7.2).

Another form of complexity already remarked upon was the variety of public agencies with a stake in action within the area. Also in the summer of 1988 central government further compounded this situation – and complemented their formal commitment to the Heartlands strategy – by winding up the Handsworth task force and switching the resources freed by this step into a new task force in East Birmingham. The area assigned to the new team goes wider than the Heartlands area, including the now largely Asian-inhabited area of Saltley, once the location of one of the earlier and largely forgotten community development projects schemes (see Chapter 2). Nevertheless, substantial overlap remains.

The intention behind the location of a task force in Nechells as described by Clarke, was to ensure that the jobs that would be attracted to the area through large-scale redevelopment would go as far as possible to local people (a key issue in Handsworth, scene of Clarke's successful battle with Cabinet colleagues to secure such priority). Emphasis was accordingly laid on skills training as well as on the promotion of small businesses. But it was difficult not to suspect a rather different intention: that the government, having decided not to invest directly in core funding for Heartlands, needed to be in a position to claim at least part of the credit for any successes that might be achieved in the area.

Implementation: the first phase

After the approval of the basic strategy, the Heartlands Board created a number of separate working parties to develop individual parts of the strategy, splitting responsibility between various interests represented on the Board, including the local authority. The general direction of the action taken, within the terms of the strategy, was determined largely by the special characteristics of the area: the opportunities, Docklands in miniature, for new development in a waterside location; close proximity to the city centre providing both opportunities and potential competition from other well-placed locations; the existence of widespread dereliction and blight, in residential as well as commercial premises; and the presence of a substantial resident population in the various neighbourhoods, with a well-established pattern of working locally but with shortages in key skills; and, finally, the issue of 'image'.

The manner of working adopted related closely to the structure of the company; as the description of its activities issued subsequently points out, it is:

> an enabling company. . . not a landowner nor a source of finance for development. . . . Its enabling role is to help create the strategic framework; to guide development in the area; to ensure its partners execute the strategy and to bring in, alongside physical developments, the various

social programmes. *In short, its aim is to bring resources or services into the area to support its regeneration.* [Emphasis added.]

(Birmingham Heartlands Ltd 1991a)

The definition of functions is crucial. Because the UDA is not itself a developer it operates almost entirely through the resources it can mobilise in other agencies, both public and private. Annual expenditure on the whole central team is only £0.6m. The status of those who sit on the Heartlands Board is a crucial factor; the fact that they are at the top of their respective organisations guarantees that approaches will not be rebuffed. The willingness of Board members to participate in working parties is also a key element in the operating style. These are task-oriented working groups, with membership and chairing related to the particular job in hand. As the statement puts it, these

provide the driving force of the initiative and are the vehicle by which detailed area-based coordination takes place. (They) bring together public and private investment in these smaller areas in a rational and coherent time frame.

(Birmingham Heartlands Ltd 1991a)

Nevertheless, the emphasis and style of approach as reflected in the documentation and on the ground varies substantially between those areas where the developers' interests are most clearly engaged and those (like estate management) where the role of the local authority is clearly more significant.

In the first category comes the 'flagship' developments, for which the key document is the Waterlinks Development Framework, billed as being 'not a masterplan but a flexible framework which aims to encourage investment and. . .guide land assembly, grant applications and planning control in the area'. The intention is to attract investment, with an emphasis on three types of development: 'flexible business space; shopping in small groups of units and leisure activities' and – with some clear exclusions – large shopping centres, warehouses and depots. Tight control over the physical form of new developments is envisaged, with a common stress on water as a feature throughout. Only a small quantity of residential provision is included; but social uses – day nurseries or 'medically related facilities' – will be considered. The outline approval of these plans has led to the preparation of a number of detailed treatments of specific sections of the canal – Aston Flight, Aston Cross and Astoria Lock – as office developments and the refurbishment of Heartlands' own headquarters, which has emerged as 'Waterlinks House'. These developments are being carried out by a separate company spun off from the main enterprise, Waterlinks plc, involving four of the five 'founder developers' (Tarmac, Wimpey, Douglas and Bryant). The first of these, Aston Flight, opened in 1990 as a 'high-tech business centre' alongside the canal, with 145,000 sq ft of office space, built in standard late 1980s postmodern style in red brick with vivid blue and red metal window frames.

The second major commercial development, the Starsite, was put out to competition in 1989. The contract for design and master plan was won by Derek Walker associates; it provides for a business exchange, with linked shopping and leisure facilities. A separate company, Starsite plc, was set up in 1990 to manage and construct the project; but progress has been held up as a result of the economic recession which began to affect the West Midlands in the same year and problems with the main site owners, Powergen. An outline planning application was expected in late 1991; but progress on the site was held up by the severity of the recession. Early in 1992, a new tactic was adopted, with the proposal that British Rail should move its central Birmingham operation from cramped and unpopular New Street station to a new location in Heartlands. This would be linked by metro to the city centre and provide an alternative focus for economic development. At the time of writing, these plans are still in the early stages of discussion.

Alongside the first two main commercial initiatives run two residential schemes, the first covering Bordesley and the second Nechells. Both have been the subject of studies, the first of these under the chairmanship of Mike Jennings, Divisional Director of Tarmac; and the second under the Chairman of Birmingham Housing Committee, Councillor Stan Austin. The areas, scheme, and general approaches differ quite widely. The Bordesley planning framework, covering an area of 95 acres with a population of 1,000 people in 350 existing dwellings, represents an attempt to establish 'a self-contained urban village with a clear and distinct identity' through construction of substantial new build schemes. These are to be undertaken by consortia of developers and, by 1991, 118 dwellings had been built by Tarmac, Wimpey and Bryant, 'the majority of which have been sold to local people'. This scheme attracted £1.4m in City Grant. Planning consent has been given for Wimpey to build a further 40 houses; and £3.7m in City Grant has been received for a 320-unit scheme by Woolwich Homes and Bellway Urban renewal. The project also includes a programme of improvements to council dwellings and should produce 600 new homes in mixed tenures by 1993. In a further phase, a village centre with shops, health facilities and a community centre will be provided (Birmingham Heartlands Ltd 1991b).

The Nechells development framework is essentially about improvements to existing local authority estates. In a long preface to the proposals, the Chairman of Birmingham Housing Committee, Stan Austin, assures his readers that 'Birmingham Heartlands has no interest whatsoever in acquiring the City's rented housing. At the end of the day decisions on City housing rest, after real consultation with tenants, with your elected representatives on the City Council and the Housing Management Committee.' Stress is placed on the importance of improving community facilities as well as upgrading housing, on restoring the image of the area and promoting equal opportunities for all its inhabitants. The obstacles are seen as shortage of funds and of manpower in the local authority and a resistance to any change ('better the devil you know'). In an area whose 2,500 houses are almost wholly in city ownership and management and which was a comprehensive development area in the 1950s acquaintance with the devil has been long and close, and the temptation to be suspicious about any new set of proposals from the same quarter is certainly strong.

However, some work has already been done on a number of the estates; there are major estate action projects to refurbish tower blocks in Duddeston Manor (£1.5m) and – notably – the Bloomsbury estate (£1.7m). This has been a DoE priority estate since 1984 and now has an Estate Management Board with executive powers and full tenant participation which has successfully launched an ambitious programme involving clearance and new construction as well as improvements (see also below, p. 159).

But generally the atmosphere on the Nechells estates (as the report correctly observes) is 'bleak and oppressive', with much scaffolding in evidence and high vacancy rates and long delays in reletting. At the time of the report (September 1989) 77 per cent of tenants were in arrears with their rent. The work being undertaken there – after a period of consultation – will involve a mixture of demolition of the least popular maisonettes and rehabilitation of the more popular tower blocks. The funding will come from a variety of sources: the city's Housing Investment Programme (much constrained), Housing Association Grant and funds from the Inner City Partnership (into whose priority area the whole of Heartlands falls).

The housing strategy for Nechells must of necessity be linked to other social issues – the lack of social facilities and support for parents of young children and the high unemployment rate, which was down to 24 per cent by late 1989 but began rising again early in 1990 (see Table 7.6). This tends to be concentrated in the 25–34 age group, with substantial long-term unemployment among older people.

The main contribution that Heartlands has made so far to addressing this problem is the support that has been given to the compact between a large group of employers extending well outside the original stakeholding developers and a group of local schools. The concept of compact originates in the United States, in Boston; it was picked up by the Inner London

Education Authority in the mid-1980s and applied in the East End of London. During his spell as Inner Cities Minister, Kenneth Clarke also came across compacts on one of his American visits and added it to the range of new devices that he vigorously promoted in a series of 'breakfast roadshows' with bankers and industrialists in major British cities (*Guardian*, 4 January 1988). The Heartlands version sets goals for performance by pupils, including attendance and involvement in work experience schemes with employers and in turn commits those employers to provide 'permanent jobs with training, or training with the assurance of a job at the end of it' to all those who meet the goals. The initial set of compacts began in 1989/90 and involve three schools (Aston Manor, Duddeston Manor and Bordesley Green) and 324 school-leavers in 1991. In 1992, the scheme extends outside Heartlands and will include seven more schools and 1,387 school-leavers. Eventually, it is intended that the compact shall become a self-sufficient agency, providing appropriate training on a city-wide basis to cover all the possible range of work for which pupils might qualify. At this point, it would be fair to say that the effectiveness of compacts as a means of enhancing the employment prospects of Heartlands school-leavers entering a highly constrained job market in deep recession has yet to be tested.

The other main area of social action is the provision of child care facilities; but on this front Heartlands itself has only a limited capacity for executive action. More significant as an area of activity has been training. The major initiative here, Joblink 2000, has been undertaken in conjunction with East Birmingham Task Force: it provides local employers with both pre-recruitment training and specific 'customised' courses after recruitment. One such scheme (twelve places) has been provided for one of Waterlinks' first tenants in Aston Cross, the Birmingham Family Health Practitioners Association. In addition, Heartlands has negotiated places for local people on a series of access schemes in FE Colleges and access centres across the city (Training Working Party: Joblink 2000).

The final-large scale initiative for which Heartlands has pressed in the initial phase of its existence has been the construction of a trunk road 3½ miles long from Junction 5 on the M6 through the area to the Dartmouth Middleway, at an estimated cost of £74m. This proposal provoked considerable local opposition, protesters arguing that it would bring both motorway and commuter traffic into the area and increase noise and pollution (*Daily News*, 9 March 1988). However, the UDA was not deterred; and an astute political campaign using the contribution that the road would make to regeneration of the area as the clinching element in the case finally persuaded the Secretary of State for Transport (Cecil Parkinson) to release funds for the project. Alongside the spine road will run the new city metro scheme, designed to provide a link from the city centre to the NEC and Birmingham Airport (see Map 7.2).

Although this project is not strictly a Heartlands initiative the benefits to the area in terms of accessibility are obvious. It also provides the focus for the third major commercial development: 'Heartlands Industrial'. This will involve a number of new initiatives. An Industrial Improvement area (IIA) came into operation in April 1990; this is intended to enhance opportunities for new industrial and business development along the spine road by providing grants for the refurbishment of property and reuse of land and premises. A number of other linked proposals have also emerged; in the Bromford area the main focus is the Fort Dunlop complex in a prominent location alongside the motorway; in Saltley, a Simplified Planning Zone (SPZ) is planned to take advantage of commercial possibilities on a number of major derelict sites (Report to Economic Development Committee, 6 November 1990).

A whole series of additional projects initiated, like the metro, by other agencies will also benefit the Heartlands area. Prominent among these are those schemes supported by the East Birmingham task force, especially in the area of skills training and child care. An ambitious attempt to bring together all the activities taking place in the area which can be broadly categorised as 'social' has recently (March 1991) been undertaken by a working party made up largely of officers from the city council's executive departments. This recommends a more closely integrated approach, based on community development within the locality and a simplified relationship to the city and existing officer groups. The main contribution likely to be made by Heartlands itself is through the establishment of a community trust. This was originally floated in the initial public consultation and was intended to come into operation once the overall strategy had been agreed. However, it did not become fully operational until June 1990 and is being funded for the moment on a small scale (the income for 1990/1 was £6,076, not all of which was spent). From this sum a number of environmental and community action projects have been funded; the trust plans to expand its activities in the near future to cover the appointment of neighbourhood community workers for the area's urban villages, with a brief to stimulate local self-help (Birmingham Heartlands Community Trust first annual report, 1991).

Progress, in sum, over the first three years of Heartlands' operation has been constrained by the uneven access to resources and shaped by the style which the Board has adopted to maximise the input from the various partner agencies and those others operating in the area. In these circumstances, any attempt at evaluation must necessarily be provisional.

ANALYSIS

What's distinctive about the UDA approach?

The broad lines along which Heartlands is likely to proceed for the next phase of its existence have now been laid down. In what ways, broadly, is the style adopted distinctive? And what impact has the form of the approach had on what has been attempted?

Before addressing this question it is important to recognise that the choice in 1987 did not lie simply between the creation of a UDC superimposed on inner Birmingham or the setting up of Heartlands in the form it finally assumed. The range of possibilities goes considerably wider. It would have been theoretically (but not politically) possible to retain the concept of a public-sector lead, either by creating a 'qualgo', a wholly-owned subsidiary of the local authority along the lines of the regional economic development agencies created by upper-tier authorities around the country in the early 1980s, or alternatively by continuing with the Inner City Partnership as the major source of funding and nesting a small area initiative within it. There was also, even in 1987, a no-change option, continuing with the crazy quilt (the image is the Audit Commission's) of local and central government schemes already in place in Birmingham – besides the Partnership, the task force and City Action Team and the various individual operations run by competing government departments, overlaid by successive layers of new ministerial bright notions and wheezes.

Perhaps most persuasive of all in the climate of 1987, a case could have been made for allowing the private sector to take an untrammelled lead, with only minimal assistance from central government, ensuring that funds flowed freely and directly to new schemes through devices like City Grant. The case made out by the CBI in their report *Initiatives Beyond Charity* suggests that with the right support such an approach would be perfectly viable. It depends upon the enlisting of the support of key local actors as individuals; but in a city like Birmingham, with its curious air of a tightly knit urban village in which 500 people are popularly supposed to 'run the city', such an approach would be perfectly feasible. An embryonic form of such an organisation already existed in the shape of a group of local businessmen calling themselves 'West Midlands United'. Moreover, the role played by the Chamber of Commerce in animating the original Heartlands proposal might also have suggested extending that approach into a wider but all-private coalition. Such an approach could also have built on the substantial involvement of a number of leading firms in the region (for example, IMI) in corporate 'social responsibility' projects (PSI Report 1991).

A little later, the *Economist*, once again acting as fugleman for the government, was to press vigorously for all-private-sector urban regeneration agencies to be included on the policy menu. These would be broadly parallel to the Training and Enterprise Councils to which the government has now entrusted the responsibility for training; they would be 'staffed by private-sector people and would charge councils and developers a fee for arranging joint ventures between them' (*Economist*, 3 June 1989). However, this argument – perhaps surprisingly – made little headway.

The argument that Birmingham City Council – with the enthusiastic support of its private sector collaborators – made to the Secretary of State in the summer of 1987 was that the UDA solution could combine the virtues of all the other different types of approach. It would deliver the goods quickly and efficiently through the direct involvement of a group of major developers, but would not be seen as an 'alien wedge' by local people, as the LDDC had been. It would not involve major start-up costs, since it could incorporate activity already under way in the area and use the networks already in place, connecting existing statutory and voluntary agencies active locally. Nor would it require a large staff to operate, since much of the work would be done by the existing departments of the local authority (which would be funded in part through existing budgets, and could be topped up where appropriate by increased allocations through the Inner City Partnership and other sources of special funding from the central government departments concerned). Essentially, it would be an enabling rather than an executive body.

But the city also went on to argue from this that despite not being in these respects a wholly new enterprise, the UDA should be treated like a UDC in being given a specific capital allocation for start-up action. The government's response was not merely to withhold such an allocation (which led one senior member of the city team to conclude that the whole enterprise had become infeasible) but also to insist that the city should undertake to behave in the planning context as if a UDC with statutory powers did exist and undertake to introduce a simplified planning regime throughout the area, which would facilitate rapid action to take full advantage of all development opportunities. The council had in fact already committed itself to a form of simplification and has had no difficulty in agreeing to the creation of simplified planning zones (SPZs) in Heartlands. But by imposing this condition the government apparently intended to dilute the local authority's detailed control over events, already weakened by the elimination of local authorities' role in the award of City Grant.

Nevertheless, despite these conditions and the predominance of the private sector both as stakeholders and as members on the Heartlands Board, the enterprise is recognisably a joint undertaking; and this is clearly reflected in the style in which it functions – the topic left entirely untouched by the consultants in their initial report. The pattern of proceeding through working parties constituted as subcommittees of the Board with joint public–private sector membership (and chairs from both sectors) has retained the collaborative flavour of the original approach. At the same time, some initiatives have been firmly placed in one camp or the other. Some development schemes lie clearly on the private side of the line and have been entrusted either to subgroups of the founder developers or hived off as separate companies (e.g. Waterlinks; Starsite). Others involving the public sector housing stock have, as far as resources permit, been left to the city to lead. Certain social programmes involving a wider group of public agencies have been brought within the scope of Heartlands by the preparation of reports by working parties. These have reviewed the activities of all the statutory agencies involved in delivering services locally (as in the report on Training, and the Social Strategy) without going to the lengths of creating formal co-ordinating machinery.

The city's role, however, remains crucial – as planning and highway authority and as housing authority. The powers attached to these functions remain in place – unlike other areas, where UDCs have been imposed; although the lack of core funding is a crucial constraint, the description in Heartlands publicity of the general approach as 'area based corporate management from the local authority supported by Heartlands Limited' is still legitimate.

Within the city bureaucracy, a standing working party was established to provide a point of entry for all requests and new policy initiatives affecting Heartlands; but this has been superseded with the arrival of a new Chief Executive by a quarterly review of progress involving chief officers. In the wider public sector arena, the support of the regional offices of central government and their directors has been crucial, both in helping to unlock resources at the disposal of the City Action Team (over which the Regional Director of DTI presided) and as advocates both in the context of the Inner City Partnership and generally. In all this activity, there has been an attempt to make a virtue out of necessity brought about by the absence of a 'core' capital grant and to aim for 'public–public' leverage of the kind that the task forces have specialised in achieving. This has been done both through the task force itself and (on a larger scale) the Inner City Partnership.

If collaboration between and within statutory agencies appears to have made good progress, there is as yet less sign of a developing statutory-voluntary relationship. This is important, since one of the key arguments has been that the feuding between the development corporation and locally-based groups that has been a constant feature of the Docklands situation would be avoided by the creation of a UDA. At the city-wide level, there has been some active cooperation – for example, with the Birmingham Voluntary Services Council and through the churches – but at local level progress has been uneven. This was partly the result of mishandling of the early stages of consultation, which generated considerable local criticism and led to the creation of an 'oppositional' Heartlands Residents Association – though this has been less in evidence more recently. It also partly reflects the slow progress on the implementation of the suggested community trust which was to have supported new community initiatives. A complicating factor more recently has been the activities of the East Birmingham task force and its energetic outreach policy, especially with the Asian community. Pressed on the question of community relations, Heartlands staff tend to talk about the passivity of the local population and the sense that they've 'seen it all before'. This sensation was certainly in evidence in BBC Midlands's review of progress in March 1990. Perhaps more damagingly, only 27 per cent of respondents questioned in the course of Birmingham Polytechnic's social survey in 1989 had any idea of what Heartlands is about and only 10 per cent felt that it would be of benefit to them (quoted in Birmingham City Council 1991).

All things considered, however, a distinctive style can be said to have emerged and is especially evident in the way in which the headquarters staff have been recruited and in their functions. By the standard of a public bureaucracy (UDCs included) this is a very small unit, made up entirely of secondees whose functions are enabling rather than line management. The total budget for staff and running costs in 1990/1 was only £500,000 – a sum met by the shareholders in proportion to their holdings (statement, February 1991). The Finance Director's success in operating in the confusing environment created by the overlapping and sometimes contradictory grant regimes operated by different government departments is a particular example of the Heartlands style, leading to effective action even if the form was determined by the restrictions originally imposed by the Secretary of State. However, the reliance on attracting specific funding for particular schemes and the absence of any capital grant that could be spent at the discretion of the agency left it dangerously exposed to the financial problems that emerged as the recession began to take hold from the beginning of 1990 and the costs associated with new development and providing satisfactory infrastructure continued to rise.

If the style is genuinely different, what tests of performance can appropriately be applied and what comparisons can be made with possible alternative forms?

How should Heartlands be evaluated?

Since actual progress on schemes is still limited, there is a strong argument for saying that any evaluation of the Heartlands UDA at this stage in its evolution is almost certain to be misleading. Even if it were possible to measure progress on a number of individual schemes, the cumulative effects of the whole operation are bound to take some years to make themselves fully felt. In the case of Docklands, it was several years from declaration before it was possible to talk with any confidence about outcomes, and six before the first comprehensive evaluations with a plausible claim to objectivity were produced (House of Commons Employment Committee 1988a and b; National Audit Office 1988). Furthermore, it can now be seen that some of the conclusions that were drawn then were premature, confusing the effects of the period of rapid growth in the national economy and consequent hyperactivity in the city with the outcome of action taken by the development corporation itself.

Nevertheless, it is in principle possible to devise a set of measures that are appropriate to the measurement of progress in an enterprise still at an early stage of development, provided that certain limitations are recognised. Firstly, there are likely to be substantial modifications in the direction and stated objectives of enterprises as those directly involved 'learn by doing' (see Spencer *et al.* 1986). Secondly, as Spencer and his colleagues point out, 'assessment of programmes may be resisted by various actors in the situation, especially those concerned more with the launching of activities than with judgments about effects' (Spencer *et al.* 1986: 165). Finally, it is important to be able to discriminate between the direct consequences of new interventions and the local effects of general regional or national trends. This problem can, it is true, be alleviated through use of comparative data – although problems of availability and selection will inevitably arise.

In the case of Heartlands, objectives have been laid down from the outset and subsequently linked to a series of implementation strategies which have in turn generated specific targets. These can be set out in tabular form (see Table 7.2)

This approach suggests that the first test that might be applied is the one favoured by the CBI (see their report *Initiatives Beyond Charity*): 'cranes on the horizon'. So, specifically, what progress has been made on new construction? In both the commercial and the residential housing sectors, a number of schemes are already on site. All schemes within the framework plans for the specific sub-areas of Heartlands are timetabled with completion dates. Measurement of this kind is therefore not merely feasible but is already being undertaken (see Table 7.3).

Table 7.2 Heartlands' objectives

Overall objectives	Main components	Specific targets (1988–98)
Attract new economic activity and jobs	Physical Development	503ha 3,696k sq ft
	Marketing Strategy	
	Investment Strategy	£1,300m
Improve living conditions for existing inhabitants	Measures directed at ensuring residents' benefit	20,000 jobs 30% increase in no. of homes

Source: Strategy document (1988) and subsequent updates

Important additional information which will become available includes lettings and sales, although as a measure of success this must be qualified by being set in the context of performance elsewhere by other broadly comparable agencies. Stoker's analysis of the style and performance of UDCs suggests that much of the commercial development in Heartlands would have been achievable by that route, although there might have been more stress on high profile schemes by some of the more 'entrepreneurial' corporations, like Teesside UDC, and perhaps less on the 'bite-sized

Table 7.3 Progress on industrial and housing developments, 1 January 1991

1. *Speculative industrial development*		
	Completed	177k sq ft
	Under construction	80k sq ft
	Planned	800k sq ft
2. *Offices*		
	Completed	60k sq ft
	Under construction	120k sq ft
3. *Housing*		
Private Sector	Under construction	118 units
	Planned	400 units
Housing Associations	Complete	60 units
	Under construction	130 units
Local Authority	Complete	480 flats
	Under construction	338 flats

Source: Progress Report, February 1991

chunks' (sic) favoured by Heartlands. When it comes to sales and lettings, any progress against the national trend in Heartlands during the current economic downturn would be especially significant. No conclusive evidence on this point is yet obtainable.

The second series of tests are the financial ones. That most commonly employed in the evaluation of urban development corporations has been 'leverage': originally, the ratio of private capital attracted through use of a corporation's core funding to those funds. This measure is not appropriate in the Heartlands case, since there is no direct core funding from the government. However, Heartlands UDA has been extremely successful in attracting different forms of grant from different 'pockets' operated by various government agencies. The clearest example is the release of £6.2m in City Grant to match £20m of money committed by private developers for Waterlinks (an unusually favourable ratio). Here, too, it is possible to produce a scoreboard, both of private sector funds committed – either directly, through the partner-developers and by 'outside' companies – and of public sector funding released by new development. This, in a slightly different sense, can also be described as a form of leverage. (A version of this is used by the local task force which claims £7m leveraged for £1.8m of direct funding; but only £0.6m of the £7m is private money – the remainder is funding from elsewhere in the public sector.)

The basic record of Heartlands at the beginning of 1991 is illustrated in Table 7.4. Of the £328.5m invested, 40 per cent is from the joint ventures of the Heartlands private shareholders, 41 per cent from other developers and 19 per cent through the City Council.

On the last item of expenditure coming through the city, there is a clear risk of double counting; and also an important issue of ownership. Since the declaration of the UDA, the city has invested heavily in schemes in Heartlands, both as part of its own main programmes and through the Inner City

Table 7.4   Heartlands' financial investment position, 1 January 1991

	Dev investment by value (£m)	Highway investment by cost (£m)
Completed since 1988	50.9	2.6
Under construction	54.2	7.4
With planning approval	131.4	108.0
Proposals under consideration	92.0	14.7
Total	328.5	132.7

Source: Progress Report, February 1991

Table 7.5 Birmingham City Council schemes in Heartlands, 1990–1

	£
1. *Partnership capital schemes*	
Economic Development Committee	1,126k
Education Committee	59k
Housing Committee	313k
Leisure Services Committee	79k
Planning Committee	211k
Social Services Committee	57k
Technical Services Committee	660k
Total	2,505k
2. *Partnership revenue schemes*	
Economic Development Committee	32k
Education Committee	4k
Leisure Services Committee	74k
Total	110k
3. *Main programme capital schemes*	
Economic Development Committee	50k
Education Committee	400k
Housing Committee	2,659k
Technical Services Committee	4,150k
Total	7,259k
Derelict Land Grants	143k
4. *Main programme revenue*	
Economic Development Committee	87k
Education Committee	211k
Housing Committee	581k
Social Services Committee	1,500k
Total	2,379k

Source: Communication from Chief Executive, 3 July 1990

Partnership. In total, this amounts to £10m for capital schemes and £2.5m in revenue in the current financial year (1990/1) (see Table 7.5 for a breakdown).

But in what sense is all this Heartlands expenditure, as opposed to expenditure which happens to have taken place in Heartlands? The federal organisational structure of the operation makes it difficult to draw a line.

Even in cases where expenditure would demonstrably not have been undertaken without the intervention of Heartlands Ltd, the administration and actual expenditure of the money obtained from the central exchequer will be the responsibility of other agencies. This is a direct consequence of the 'enabling' role played by Heartlands which contrasts sharply with existing UDCs with their substantial budgets and wider executive functions and makes comparison with their track record difficult. The main argument for the Heartlands approach in this context is that by 'making the case and setting the strategic framework', developments have been made possible which would not have occurred if an independent corporation had been functioning in the area – or if individual developers had been acting on their own account. Looking at the breakdown of schemes, it is difficult not to conclude that one decisive factor has been the existence of the Partnership and the willingness of partner agencies to give Heartlands some degree of priority, as they have done since the 1988/91 Partnership planning round.

These difficulties do not arise in the case of the limited number of schemes funded directly by Heartlands UDA from its own limited budget. In particular, a useful measure of activity on social and community action will be the amount of funding allocated to the community trust when this is finally set up in independent form, and the categories of scheme supported.

A third category of measure may also help, based on the local resident population. There is, after all, no ambiguity about the boundaries of the Heartlands area: people either live or work within it or they do not. The consultants' (Tym 1987a) report provides baseline data about the circumstances of residents at the time of submission (November 1987). This has been usefully updated by the Birmingham Polytechnic's social survey (carried out in 1988) which is particularly helpful in pinpointing a number of changes that have taken place. These have been particularly notable in age structure, with substantial increases in the numbers of under-15s, ethnic composition – with a growth in the Afro-Caribbean population, which now comprises 30 per cent of the population, as compared to 13 per cent Asian and 43 per cent UK-born – and in increased numbers of single-parent households headed by women. The polytechnic's linked survey of financial circumstances (1990) underlines the extent of the problems of poverty that affect the area: for example, only 23 per cent of respondents reported that they were debt-free – not a surprising finding, given that 62 per cent of all households were living on less than £100 per week (Birmingham City Council 1991).

Basic demographic information can give some indication of the development of Heartlands and the impact of action taken since declaration. Even the size of the local population can be a relevant indicator, either as a surrogate for activity – housing clearances – or for state of morale. Ethnic composition is also often, and controversially, used as a proxy for the extent of deprivation. Other measures are routinely used as indicators of 'malaise', or whatever term is currently fashionable (there is a huge literature on this topic, much of it illustrating how difficult it is to achieve objective measurement). There is also a practical difficulty with using census-based measures in intercensal years.

Latterly, however, the tendency has been to rely on one measure as a proxy: the unemployment rate, now routinely obtainable down to ward level on a monthly basis. In the second annual review of the totality of the government's inner city initiatives, the main indicator of the success provided was the fall in unemployment in the target areas (Department of the Environment 1990b: 5). However, this figure is wholly meaningless without direct comparisons with national, regional and local trends (needless to say, these were not provided). As unemployment rates have now turned up again nationally, it is a safe bet that this indicator will not be prominent in the next review report. Nevertheless, unemployment rates are an important indication of the economic health of a neighbourhood, especially when part of the local population is employed within the Heartlands area itself. Over a longer timespan, the unemployment measure – set in context – can be a useful indicator of the extent of economic progress, to the extent that it benefits the local population (see Table 7.6).

Progress on employment can be assessed in another way, in terms of job creation. This is an area in which Heartlands has a specific objective: the creation of 20,000 new jobs. Two issues arise here: firstly, how far the jobs created go directly to local people; and secondly, the extent to which they are generated by displacement of activity from other areas. In other words, is the job gain net or gross, city-wide? The evaluation of the Handsworth task force (PA/Cambridge Economic Consultants 1991b) suggests that this can be achieved: the consultants were able to provide measures both of the extent to which new jobs benefited local inhabitants (94 per cent of them

Table 7.6 Ward-level unemployment rates for Heartlands, 1988–91

	%						
	June 88	*Jan 89*	*June 89*	*Jan 90*	*June 90*	*Jan 91*	*April 91*
Aston Ward	27.6	25.2	22.5	22.5	20.8	22.2	24.2
Nechells Ward	27.9	24.7	22.1	20.7	18.9	20.7	23.1
Birmingham	15.4	13.3	11.4	10.9	10.3	11.5	12.9

Source: WMEB Monthly Returns

went to locals) and members of ethnic minorities (who obtained 69 per cent) and of the extent to what they term 'additionality' – they estimate that between 69 per cent and 79 per cent of jobs and training places were genuinely new and that only 10–25 per cent could be clearly attributed to 'displacement' from other areas. However, a further evaluation of the task forces from the same source suggests that the effects may have been ephemeral. The authors comment:

> Only 32 per cent of projects have continued on at full strength to maintain the economic momentum which the Task Force had built up. Task Force benefits in Handsworth are therefore fading away quite quickly and the cumulative total of benefits is moving onto a plateau. The main reason for this is that the capacity of local organisations and large 'flagship' projects had not been established when the Task Force closed.
>
> (PA/Cambridge Economic Consultants 1991b)

The authors add that 'the lessons of Handsworth have been learned'. Clearly there are also important implications for Heartlands, in terms of sustaining support, once given.

Alongside measures of jobs created, with these clarifications go places on schemes. Here again, the involvement of Heartlands UDA in a number of new initiatives provides an apparently straightforward measure of performance. The educational compact would be a clear example of such a scheme, where ownership is not in doubt. However, with the first cohort of school-leavers not yet fully in the job market, it is too early to draw any conclusions. Other schemes will be more complex to assess; and the activities of the East Birmingham task force will also be a complicating factor. Their targets are very simply expressed, in terms of jobs created, training places and business schemes supported; yet their activities overlap (and in one case at least combine) with those of Heartlands and other agencies. One example is the important skills audit conducted by PE/Inbucon, which has helped to define the extent of the training task confronting all the agencies active in the area. Allocating credit in this (and other) cases without double counting looks like a potentially formidable undertaking.

Other indicators of activity specific to the Heartlands area or its inhabitants include measures of housing quality and health. In an area where local authority housing is overwhelmingly the dominant tenure, information about housing conditions and vacancies and lettings is accessible and relevant (see for example Birmingham Heartlands Ltd 1989b). Changes in these will both be significant in their own right for what they have to say about housing circumstances, and will also provide some guidance on morale in the local community. Similarly with health, where the Central District Audit of three years ago identified some important deficiencies in provision, with only two day nurseries and one health centre and no proper day centres for the elderly, and a clear need for better preventive services.

The final area of evaluation is the least tangible of all, but is related directly to one of the major goals of Heartlands, as defined both in the original consultants' report and subsequently: the enhancement of the image of the area. Much of the expenditure, both on publicity and on visual enhancement of the area (e.g. the 'gateways'; the conditions attached to Waterlinks developments), is directed to this end. The extent of success here is likely to be difficult to measure. One simple test will be the commercial one: how the pattern of sales and lettings of new development progresses.

Yet, as London Docklands has dramatically illustrated, a national economic downturn can severely damage the prospects of even the most apparently promising local schemes. *Equally*, setbacks at regional level – the interruption from 1990 of Birmingham's earlier recovery from deep recession and the resulting economic pressures – has inhibited firms (both national and international) from investing locally. The marketing of the high-profile prestige project, Starsite, was held back as a result of these developments and its role in the promotion of Heartlands has been downgraded. A catty account of the state of play in the autumn of 1990 in the *Economist* laid particular stress on the problems that this would present, commenting, 'no wonder Heartlands has run into trouble trying to pay both for cleaning up its poisoned star site, plagued by underground gas pipes and electric cables, and for relocating lots of messy scrap-yards' (*Economist*, 27 October 1990).

Another measure of image will be in the political arena. This is an area in which Heartlands already claims a substantial measure of success. The bipartisan commitment of the city council is undoubted and apparently secure, though it might not survive a leftward shift in the Labour group of the kind that took place in Manchester. The possible backlash against concentration on a specific area to the possible detriment of others similarly circumstanced has not yet materialised: even the shift in emphasis away from Handsworth has passed apparently without public protest despite the presence of a substantial group of black councillors on the Labour side. This may be partly attributable to careful cultivation of back-bench ward councillors in the area by the Heartlands team.

Nationally, the major factor appears to be a real shift in the attitude of central government towards collaborative ventures. Nicholas Ridley has left both the DoE and the government; but even before his departure a shift in attitudes was detectable. David Hunt (as Minister for Local Government) was positively enthusiastic about Heartlands' prospects, as was Alan

Howarth (junior Minister with responsibility for East Birmingham task force). Some of this is attributable to personalities: a key factor was the appointment of Reginald Eyre as Chairman. With his unrivalled set of links within the Conservative party made through holding ministerial office (and as a whip) Sir Reginald is an emollient bipartisan figure on the local scene; he also has his own priorities for action which he has set out in a Conservative political centre pamphlet: he is not by any means simply a figurehead.

Some of this stems from substantial amendments in the Conservative government's overall position towards local government – a change measurable in terms of difference in tone between *Action for Cities* and *People in Cities* two years later. This may partly be due to a belated perception that UDCs are not quite the surefire bet that Patten and others thought they were in the different circumstances of 1987, and partly to the criticisms of their earlier position (cf. Audit Commission report of 1989: 'nothing is likely to have a greater adverse effect on the private sector's perception of an area than evidence of disunity between two branches of the public sector') and some to changes in the attitudes of local authorities themselves. An important additional factor in Birmingham has been strong positive messages going 'up the line' to Whitehall from the regional directors of DTI and DoE/Department of Transport. Reconciliation was sealed by Dick Knowles's knighthood, evidence of ministers' perception that he was a local authority leader with whom they could do business.

If there is any risk of disruption of Heartlands' progress as a result of the Conservative government's activities it seemed until recently likely to come as an unintended consequence of other policy initiatives. An example would be the recent creation of the Training and Enterprise Councils (TECs) and the effect that this may have on training budgets and priorities in the city and hence in the Heartlands area, or other new actors appearing on the scene as a result of policy initiatives in housing and education not directly related to inner city policy but impacting upon it. However, any complacency was rudely disturbed by the city council's failure in the City Challenge organised by Michael Heseltine (July 1991) in which the city had put forward a scheme in East Birmingham, based in part in the Heartlands (Bordesley) and using as a basis many of the devices successfully employed in Heartlands. Given that one of the major themes of City Challenge, as set out in the guidance documentation, was intended to be the promotion of the role of local government as a leader in building up collaborations with central government and other local interests, this failure was particularly unfortunate. Quite apart from depriving the city of access to much-needed resources to promote further activities locally, it seemed to suggest that the apparent fit between the Heartlands-declared objectives and those of the City Challenge exercise had gone unrecognised by DoE ministers.

Nevertheless, generally improved relations with central government would not be disturbed by a change of government nationally. The concept of public–private sector collaboration in urban regeneration is wholly consistent with the general lines adopted in the Labour Party's policy review (which states baldly that UDCs will be 'brought under democratic control') and more recent (1991) policy statements.

The final and in some ways most important area in which image may be crucial is in relation to the confidence of the local population. Promotion of their interests through direct involvement has featured in the various versions of the strategy from the outset. Their initial response has already been referred to; although outright hostility was of comparatively short duration, reservations clearly persist and were expressed in the BBC Midlands television report of March 1990 and the subsequent social survey (quoted above) which also reflected strong dissatisfaction with living conditions in the area, lack of job opportunities, levels of crime and 'inadequate policing' (quoted in Birmingham City Council 1991).

Some attempts have been made from the outset to deliver on this objective. There has been a strong emphasis on consultation on specific schemes; and the housing developments have been the subject of detailed exercises in which tenant choice was not merely taken into account but, in one case at least, decisive. Heartlands staff includes a community liaison worker – a former Labour councillor with strong local connections, well aware of the problems that an over-simple approach to community consultation may throw up, especially for developing working relationships with ethnic minorities.

Apart from supporting these activities, Heartlands have also tried to move beyond the rather rigid model of consultation employed (plan-and-public meeting) in launching the original strategy – an approach which clearly proved to be deficient in securing the confidence of locals. The clearest example of this process at work has been the encouragement given to the Bloomsbury Estate Management Board. This grew out of the Priority Estate Project (PEP) established by the DoE on the Bloomsbury estate in 1984; it consists of twelve elected tenants, four Council nominees and four co-opted members. The Board has housing management powers and controls its own revenue budget; the city retains property ownership. The Board proposed in November 1990 a full-scale redevelopment scheme for the estate, put it out to consultation (achieving a response rate of a little over one-half of the households on the estate, who broadly supported the approach proposed) and enlisted a consortium of housing associations to implement the scheme. As a model of participation, this is a radical departure from the passive consultation of earlier phases, although Heartlands is the location for the scheme rather than the driving force behind it.

Despite these and other innovations – e.g. the provision of community-based facilities – the UDA is still potentially vulnerable to a determined effort by a credible local opposition group to attack its credentials as an agency that genuinely has the interests of the local inhabitants at heart. The example of Docklands is instructive here, too; the long campaign waged by the Docklands Consultative Committee against the objectives and priorities of the LDDC looks far more credible now than it did during the Lawson Boom and it may well be a crucial influence in determining whether Docklands survives a change of government (if it occurs) and continues as a UDC to the end of its scheduled existence in 1996.

Reliance on surveys of local opinion and audits of customer satisfaction may help to build bridges; but the key test is likely to be delivery on undertakings given to local people like those in Councillor Austin's Preface to the Nechells Development Plan. The social strategy for Heartlands, prepared in the Spring of 1991, identifies an important gap in the range of activities in Heartlands and deficiencies in the style in which they are undertaken. The authors prescribe a strong dose of decentralised community development to make good both deficiencies – with what result, if any, remains to be seen.

CONCLUSIONS

The central issue around the organisational form of the Heartlands UDA was whether the looser, enabling format, with a small central staff, heavy reliance on both public and private partner agencies to provide the executive action and extensive use of working parties to determine the form of action was more efficient than the 'singlemindedness' of the UDCs. For some purposes, the Heartlands model seemed to work very effectively; but the absence of core grant posed problems in addressing major developments like Starsite – especially in recession conditions.

In fact, it was this absence of a significant capital resource that eventually led the Heartlands Board and Birmingham City Council to seek and receive a change of status to that of urban development corporation. This was agreed by the Secretary of State, Michael Heseltine, in January 1992 and received the approval of the House of Commons by affirmative order just before the 1992 General Election. The new Heartlands UDC will have a life span of five years. At first sight, this switch in status appears to negate many of the principles established in the course of the lifespan of the Heartlands UDA. However, in practice the changes arising from the change of status are less drastic than might appear. Although there is a surrendering of direct control to the centre in return for a fixed capital allocation (£50m per year for five years) the form of the UDC itself is to be very different to that of the earlier Mark II UDCs. The existing chairman of Heartlands UDA, Sir Reginald Eyre, retains his position; and the Leader of Birmingham City Council (Sir Dick Knowles) becomes vice-chairman. Six members of the Board will come from the local authority, matching an equivalent number from the private sector (though these cannot now include representatives of the original Heartlands group of developers, who will have to drop out as a result of their direct financial interest in developments). This is a marked departure from previous practice, in which local authority representatives have always been in a small minority. The Heartlands emphasis on balanced programmes with a strong social element will remain, as will the more flexible style of working. The Development Corporation has adopted the Development Strategy in the form that Heartlands UDA devised it; and the new chief executive of the Development Corporation will be the former deputy chief executive of Heartlands Ltd. Central government control will be exercised through the DoE regional office, which has been sympathetic from the outset to the objectives of the UDA. In sum, Heartlands philosophy and practice will continue – although the new arrangement does represent a departure from the original principle of cooperation directly entered into at the local level.

On the content of programmes, following Robson (Robson 1988), we could identify the following dangers which might result from developments in Heartlands – even if some or most of them are successful, by the measures identified in the previous section:

a) 'Jobless growth'
b) Branchplant syndrome
c) Neglect of social dimension.

On (a), 'Jobless growth', it is already clear that jobs will be generated in Heartlands. In the first phase, they will be predominantly in the construction industry, then in the office and specialist retail sectors. The skills audit undertaken in the wider East Birmingham task force area reveals a severe shortage of relevant skills in all these categories (PE/Inbucon 1989). Even where they exist, there is also a chronic shortage of support facilities – principally child-minding (Birmingham Voluntary Services Council 1989). The issue of local preference for jobs is on the policy agenda, but it will be difficult to sustain unless the skill profile is dramatically improved and more precisely targeted to the types of job that will become available. So key areas of action (and evaluation) must be the compact and its success, and the joint activities with the East Birmingham task force in promoting training (as, for example, with 'Just For Starters' and Joblink 2000). A complicating factor is the circumstances of Asian women, who are having difficulty in locating work that takes account of their special social and cultural needs. Some special programmes are being put in place to deal with this situation, but their scope may need extending. In summary, the risk seems to be not so much jobless growth as some real growth in new jobs but inaccessibility to the locals of all but the most basic service jobs.

On (b), Branchplant syndrome, the danger seems to be less significant than in 'greenfield' UDCs. Japanese companies are entering the West Midlands scene in substantial numbers; but despite the brave words in the Roger Tym report on accessibility to motorway network and airport, they do not seem likely to be tempted into Heartlands when they have Telford at their full disposal. If they do come, they are likely to generate a fair number of 'screwdriver' jobs for young workers (of both genders) and older women assembling high-tech consumer goods; the proximity of Aston Science Park might be an incentive here, although the Japanese do not seem at present to be looking for life at the technological leading edge. Nor, more to the point, is there all that much capacity in Heartlands for large-scale operations of this kind. Likelier incomers are head offices of large businesses (banking, insurance, accountancy practices, general white-collar business sector) relocating from London. Here, Robson's warning about surrendering economic control to London as command centre may be more relevant.

Neglect of the social dimension, however, is crucial to longer-term success, as the authors of the Social Strategy are at pains to stress. The lessons of Docklands for this area have been learned; and the UDA's ability both to mobilise city resources directly and influence the style in which they are delivered (as with Nechells Development Strategy) ought to have been a particular strength here. But Heartlands' identification with the previous performance of city agencies is not an unmixed blessing – in particular, past failures in housing are still a large item on the debit side. Nor will it be possible to wash out the problem with increased public expenditure. The funding of the housing programme is already a patchwork, and the city's direct contribution is unlikely to be higher than the 1990/1 allocation and may well have to be lower. With the HIP allocation at its lowest-ever level and the impact of loss of revenue to the city through the poll tax débâcle, future prospects in this sector are bleak. Whether it will be possible to leverage more from the private sector (the Housing Corporation currently has its own problems, though promised jam tomorrow) is a question that needs pressing.

Robson also makes the point that there are limits to the effectiveness of civic boosting, especially with a cacophony of competing claims being broadcast simultaneously to prospective clients, at home and abroad. But in the start-up stage some hype is inevitable. The test here is whether a distinctive identity can be created which is more than a logo and a lick of paint. This would have to incorporate rather than exclude (compare Docklands again) those locals who should be among the main – but not the only – beneficiaries and not undermine their sense of belonging to the neighbourhoods that provide the real social cement. This is where the major prestige projects – Starsite, Waterlinks – are particularly important. If, despite achieving commercial success, they become symbols of a new identity that excludes – literally in the sense of generating jobs and profits that go elsewhere – then the image of Heartlands as a 'glittering shroud' for Aston and Nechells may become only too appropriate.

8 Private enterprise alone

The manipulative (or interventionist) component of the enterprise strategy – the use of incentives to attract investment to areas where it would not otherwise go – incurs public costs in the form of tax income foregone and the more direct costs of providing infrastructure. There will be occasions, however, when the same end of increased investment in or near to inner city areas can be achieved at little or no public expense. They will, it must be admitted, be largely fortuitous, depending as they do on circumstances (usually ownership of land) which make development feasible without benefit of subsidy or incentive. The potential for such unlevered development which will have an impact on inner city areas is an unknown quantity (and will vary over time depending on the state of the market, the perceived profitability of such development schemes and so on) but it may be very considerable. Indeed, the amount of unsubsidised potential development may exceed the total volume of investment that may be expected to be levered into designated inner city areas.

It may appear at first sight that a largely unquantifiable amount of development in or near to inner city areas (whether designated or not) would only be of interest in so far as it contributed to local economic activity. It would appear to be of little import for inner city policy in any direct way. Yet this need not necessarily be true, as the example described later in this chapter will demonstrate. The potential value (for inner city policy) of unlevered, fortuitous developments lies in the fact that rarely if ever are they 'pure private'. All will require local planning permission and very large developments (such as the proposal examined here) are liable to be 'called in' by the Secretary of State and may be subject to a planning inquiry. Local planning authorities, in granting planning permissions, will almost always impose some requirements and conditions (in respect of road layouts, landscaping and so on) and the Secretary of State will almost certainly do so in relation to permissions given. And along the way, local planning authorities and developers will, between them, have entered all kinds of compromises on a range of issues. The point is that local planning authorities are not passive spectators of development schemes; they can, and do, influence a number of aspects of any development plan but this is not usually thought of in terms of potential benefit to inner cities. But there are a number of things that local authorities can do both to influence the nature of developments themselves or – more importantly – to exploit development for the benefit of inner city residents. The latter holds very considerable potential but has not been pursued with energy. Indeed, it seems that the more automatic response of many planning authorities to the possibility of large-scale development in any proximity to the inner city (or, perhaps, what they really fear, the city centre) is to refuse planning permission rather than to calculate what gain they can wring from it for the benefit of inner city areas.

In this chapter we look at one development proposal which had the potential to be exploited for inner city gain. The proposal has not yet come to fruition (for reasons that will become clear) and we are not in a position to say what form this exploitation would (as opposed to could) have taken. But when we come, in Chapter 9, to evaluate the impact on the inner cities of the enterprise strategy, we shall examine the variety of methods that could be used by local authorities to extract benefit from schemes such as this. In this chapter we shall confine ourselves to providing a sketch of the proposed scheme and the context in which it was located, both spatially and strategically.

The example we use is of particular relevance to our study of the enterprise strategy because the 'inner city issue' was at the forefront of the arguments about whether planning permission should be granted. The proposed scheme was subject to a public inquiry and in consequence a large volume of data was generated about it, about a number of kindred proposals, the urban context in which they were situated, and about likely or potential impact on inner city areas, retail centres, the environment and so on. We use the example of the Trafford Centre to examine some of the planning issues that surround the proposed development of a very large 'pure private' scheme which is so located as to have the potential to affect inner city areas for good or bad. In the course of our analyses, we shall draw heavily on evidence, arguments, and data that were prepared for and presented at the planning inquiry into the desirability or otherwise of granting planning permission to this and a number of other schemes in the same area. It behoves us therefore to enter a caveat about these data and arguments.

Planning inquiries are strange events. Similar to our legal system, they are adversarial, with interested parties (the developers, local authorities, the local butterfly society) wheeling on witnesses to present evidence to support their own case or cast opprobrium on others'. The same data are often used to support exactly opposing viewpoints. Rather like academics debating but with one fundamental difference: in planning inquiries there is the informed adjudicator: the Inspector. It is the Inspector's job to weigh the evidence and come to a judgement and this involves not only balancing arguments but also determining whether the data say what the witnesses have said they say. Most of the data we cite in subsequent paragraphs are 'agreed data': that is, data that all parties in the inquiry accept as non-disputable. (The fun comes in how witnesses use the information of course.) None the less, this is an adversarial process and it is not a witness's job to present all sides of an argument. The information they use therefore will be selective (even if 'agreed'). We have attempted to extract from the evidence put to the inquiry (some 2 million words is a conservative estimate) those data and arguments that are relevant to the potential impact of the Trafford Centre on inner city areas nearby. In this chapter we confine ourselves to outlining the relevant arguments about inner city impact and presenting the information that is necessary to evaluate this impact. The evaluation itself we present in Chapter 9 as part of our wider evaluation of the 'reach' of private enterprise.

THE TRAFFORD CENTRE

Between July 1986 and April 1987, the Manchester Ship Canal Company submitted a number of outline planning applications to Trafford Metropolitan Borough Council[1] to develop a sub-regional shopping centre and a regional sports complex on land that it owns at Dumplington on the borders of Trafford and Salford, some 3½ miles from the boundary of Manchester (see Map 5.1, p. 74). The whole site is within the designated area of the Trafford Park Development Corporation established in 1987, but all the groundwork and preparation for the proposal had been done before the corporation's designation and was not dependent upon its designation in any way.

The entire site (to be known as the Trafford Centre) consisted of some 304 areas approximately equally divided between the shopping centre and the sports complex. The shopping centre was to prove to be a more contentious proposal than the sports complex, not least because of its size (some 1m sq ft of retail floorspace)[2] but also because it was one of a number of retail centre proposals in the air at the time in the western sector of the Greater Manchester Conurbation, all part of the boom in 'out-of-town' shopping which in hindsight probably peaked in the mid 1980s and has declined since. Most of what we have to say about the Trafford Centre therefore will concern the proposal for the shopping centre.

The Trafford Centre was to be a large development by any standards (see Table 8.1) – as large, in fact, as the entire Heartlands development area (see Chapter 7) – and being situated so close to the inner areas of the conurbation (and to several city centres) its potential impact, both in terms of inner city areas and existing centre-city retailing, was sufficient in itself for the proposal to be put under close scrutiny. In fact, almost all applications for developments in excess of 250,000 sq ft are 'called in' by the Secretary of State, and as we have noted there were four other substantial (and a number of smaller)[3] applications in the pipeline (mainly for retail development) in the conurbation. The Secretary of State called in the applications under Section 35 of the Town and Country Planning Act 1971 and ordered a public inquiry, to be held in two parts: a Plenary Inquiry to consider conurbation-wide issues raised by the five major applications, and a Sector Inquiry to consider individual applications in the context of the sector of the conurbation in which they fell. (All five applications mentioned above fell into the western sector of the conurbation at varying distances from the conurbation centre.)

The Plenary Inquiry was held between 22 September and 28 October 1987 and the Salford/Trafford Sector Inquiry between 3 November 1987 and 26 February 1988. The Inspectors' Reports to both inquiries were issued in August 1989 along with the responses of the Secretary of State. So far as the Trafford Centre was concerned, the Inspector at the Sector Inquiry recommended that it be given planning permission, but the Secretary of State, on the basis of information received *after* the inquiries from the Department of Transport concerning possible congestion on the M63 motorway resulting from the scheme, declined to determine the application.

Table 8.1   Trafford Centre: Shopping centre approximate floor areas by use

Approximate Floor Space in Square Feet	
Shop units and department stores	1,000,000
Mall	146,300
Administration, public toilets and other circulation	43,000
Restaurant	9,700
Gourmet hall	28,000
Children's world	30,100
Food court	26,900
Multiplex cinema	39,800
Approximate Total Floor Area	1,323,800

Source: Manchester Ship Canal Company, Outline Planning Application: The Trafford Centre, 1 April 1987 (Manchester Ship Canal Company 1987)

What has happened since is of only peripheral interest to our concern with inner cities, but we shall, for the sake of completeness (and because the issue is still 'live'), conclude the chapter with a brief summary of developments since late 1989.

THE LOCAL CONTEXT

The Trafford Centre is an example *par excellence* of what we have called 'pure private' investment that would have had (and may still have) an important impact on inner city areas. It is located in an urban development corporation designated area, and close to large parts of the economic and social problem areas identified in the Greater Manchester Structure Plan (Greater Manchester Council 1986: G1, G2), and lies on the doorstep of the Manchester/Salford Partnership area and other large undesignated tracts of inner city deprivation (see Map 5.1 on p. 74). In this key location, the Manchester Ship Canal Company were prepared to invest some £150m without benefit of public subsidy.

The Trafford Centre site is located in Dumplington within what was the Trafford Park industrial estate, an area of some 1,267 hectares developed at the turn of the century to provide the best possible operating environment for local firms (Trafford Park Investment Strategy 1986: 5). It was, in its day, a model industrial estate but since the late 1950s it has been in steady decline, with loss of economic activity and jobs and a serious deterioration in its environment to the point where vast tracts of land are characterised by dereliction. The Park has traditionally provided employment for workers from Trafford, Salford and Manchester including the inner areas of all three (Stocks 1987b: 48), but in the twenty years from 1965 it lost more than 50 per cent of its workers (from 52,000 in 1965 to 24,500 in 1985) (Trafford Park Investment Strategy 1986: 3). Between 1983 and 1986 there was a further drop of 5 per cent (Trafford Park Investment Strategy 1986: 3). It was largely in response to this decline, and following publication of the Trafford Park Investment Strategy (TPIS) prepared by a group of five consultants, that the decision was taken to designate the Park (and some additional land on the north bank of the Manchester Ship Canal) as an urban development corporation in 1987 (see Chapter 5).

The Manchester Ship Canal Company proposal therefore would appear to be an ideal scheme for consideration, even if it did not conform exactly with what the TPIS strategy, and subsequently the development corporation, had in mind for the Dumplington site:[4] one million sq ft of retail space providing some 6,500 jobs in an Urban Development Corporation and with no leverage costs. This however was not the case, and in many respects the nature of the opposition to the proposal from a number of proximate local authorities illustrates much of what we have said in earlier chapters about the tyranny of area designations. We shall not be concerned here with the counter arguments to the Trafford Centre put by proponents of 'competing' schemes who gave evidence at the inquiries – they had rather specific interests to defend.[5] The nature of the objections of some local authorities however are worth surveying because of the more general issues they raised. In total, nine local authorities gave evidence at the inquiries, though seven of these formed a consortium because their views were similar and all objected to all the proposals in question. These seven authorities were:

Tameside Borough Council
Manchester City Council
Bolton Borough Council
Wigan Borough Council
Oldham Borough Council
Bury Borough Council
Rochdale Borough Council

The other two authorities were Trafford Borough Council and Salford City Council. By including these authorities and excluding the evidence adduced on behalf of other developers, we do not imply that the former were not *parti pris* whilst the latter were. All the authorities to some extent had their own axe to grind (and in particular, Trafford and Salford) but their objections and endorsements were based on a wider view of events and – of particular relevance here – often focused on the inner city issue.

The views of authorities other than those in the consortium were of course coloured by the locations of the various schemes. The Trafford Centre site, as we have seen, is located within the boundaries of Trafford as also is the site of one of the other very large schemes proposed by Prudential Insurance at Carrington. The third very large scheme by Fee and Company was to be located at Barton Locks within Salford but close to its boundary with Trafford. The question for Salford was whether it wanted a large retail development (which the Regatta Centre at Barton Locks was also to be) within its boundaries at all. If it did, then there was no alternative to the Barton Locks development, and since it was almost a certainty that only one large retail development would get approval (if any did) this would entail objecting to the Trafford Centre. That is the strategy that Salford adopted. The Salford Rule 6 Statement (prepared in accordance with the Town and Country Planning (Inquiries Procedure) Rules 1974), in which it outlined its arguments for the Barton Locks proposal and its objections to other proposals (including the Trafford Centre), laid much stress on the contribution that the Barton Locks development would make to inner city regeneration in Salford. The authority, the statement argued, had a well-known commitment to urban regeneration and 'Provision of a large new shopping centre at Barton Locks is a major extension of this process' (Salford 1987a: para 5.2). Furthermore, 'Urban regeneration requires positive planning for investment in locations *within or in proximity to the major concentrations of urban deprivation*' (Salford 1987a: para. 5.2; emphasis added).

Similar arguments could have been made equally about the Trafford Centre, but that was in Trafford, and for reasons we have noted, if Barton Locks was to be promoted, then the Trafford Centre would have to have been the subject of objections. There was one further inner city string to the Salford bow. The authority had collaborated with Fee and Company over the Barton Locks development and was happy to argue in its Rule 6 Statement that

> The Fee proposal therefore holds out the prospect of a genuine partnership between the public and the private sector which will be of practical assistance to the implementation of a comprehensive restructuring and radical improvement of the older urban areas of the City.
>
> (Salford 1987a: para 5.7)

This might have turned out to be a Heartlands in miniature (see Chapter 7) but the Inquiry Inspector recommended that preference be given to the Trafford Centre scheme, and the Secretary of State has concurred in this, though at the same time not ruling out the possibility of permission for the Fee proposal.

Salford objected to the Trafford Centre on a number of grounds, none of which appear entirely convincing. The first echoed the preferred use for the Dumplington site on the part of the development corporation. A retail scheme on this site, Salford argued, 'would not produce the optimum pattern of land use to further the important objective of regeneration' (Salford 1987b: para 11.1b), and that this purpose would be better served by a science or business park. No explanation was given however for why a science or business park would better aid the process of regeneration than a large retail centre and, given the arguments we have adduced in Chapter 4, it is difficult to see what the logic could be. The second objection seems even less forceful. The Barton Locks site, it was argued, lay 'outside but in close proximity to: the Assisted Area, the Partnership Area, the Enterprise Zone and the Urban Development Area' and would 'support a major new shopping centre without any of the financial and other benefits associated with special status' (Salford 1987a: para 11.1b), by which is meant, presumably, without the costs of the incentives that apply in special status areas. Yet all of these points applied equally well to the Trafford Centre site; indeed, it lies closer to major areas of deprivation than does Barton Locks and, although situated in the development corporation area, would also have incurred no incentives costs. (The third main objection was only indirectly related to inner city matters. It was that the Trafford Centre would irretrievably damage Salford's Retail Strategy which we must assume included the promotion of the Fee scheme.)

One further objection to the Trafford Park Scheme was made by the Chief Technical Services Officer for Salford at the Sector Inquiry. It was that the Dumplington site was of strategic importance both in terms of its position in the development corporation and as the only remaining large greenfield site in the conurbation suitable for use as a business or technology park which, as we have noted, were the preferred uses of the Corporation itself (Struthers 1987: paras 7.15–7.19). However, elsewhere in his evidence in promoting the Barton Locks Scheme, Mr Struthers, citing the Metro Centre in Gateshead, argued that such large retail developments were best suited to the employment needs of the inner cities. Though he does not elicit the point in his evidence, what seems to be at issue here is a prioritisation of land uses. On the one hand, a good case can be made that a large-scale retail centre would produce more employment benefit for inner city residents than would a high technology science park. On the other hand, if such a park were needed (for whatever reason) and Dumplington were the only suitable site, then clearly its use for this purpose would have to be given serious consideration. The dilemma is then complicated by the fact that the preferred use as a science park was a part of the strategy of the development corporation itself – an instrument claimed by the government to be at the forefront of inner city regeneration (Trafford Park Development Corporation 1987). Clearly, not all the development in the corporation's designated area could be for retail purposes (indeed, to promote this would not maximise employment benefit to the inner cities), but this conflict of potential land use does raise the question of whether regenerating a large industrial estate like Trafford Park is the best or most effective way of reducing urban deprivation. We shall return to this in a subsequent chapter.

The position of Trafford Borough Council in respect of the Trafford Centre was made more complicated by the fact that two large retail proposals were on offer within its boundaries, as well as a third somewhat smaller scheme at Barton Dock Road. Both officers and members in Trafford were agreed that the inner city issue was the major one in deciding on the Trafford Centre, but they were not as one about whether *any* development ought to be allowed and disagreed about whether, if there were to be any, it should be at the Carrington or Dumplington sites. There were of course many considerations besides the impact on the inner cities that had to be taken into account, not least among them the impact on existing city, sub-regional and local shopping provision, environmental impact, greenbelt policy and transportation matters. But it was inner city impact that proved to be pivotal. In order to make better sense of the various strands to the arguments put to the inquiry on behalf of Trafford Borough Council (but confining our coverage to matters relating to the inner city), we shall summarise briefly the content of the evidence put by the Chief Planning Officer to both Plenary and Sector Inquiries, review the evidence of the Chairman of the Planning Committee and finally outline the Rule 6 depositions in respect of both the Trafford Centre and the Carrington Schemes.

In evidence to the Plenary Inquiry, the purpose of which was to cast an overview of the impact of all the schemes and not to promote any one over the others (a discipline that not all witnesses were able to cope with), the Chief Planning Officer considered the case in relation to inner city impact of the Trafford Centre, the Barton Locks Scheme and the Carrington proposal. He was careful not to be selective between the three but was able to show that a case could be made for any one of them. There were differences in job generation and net job gain between the schemes but any one of the three could be justified, he argued, on the grounds that similar levels of job gain available to inner city residents simply could not be achieved in any proximate city centre, if only because no site of a suitable size was available and that achieving the same job growth in small increments within any city centre was not a feasible alternative (Stocks 1987a: 3.7–3.11).[6] Furthermore, Stocks noted that all three schemes had the potential to meet the policy aims of the *Action for Cities* strategy and would do so without incurring public sector costs by way of inducements (Stocks 1987a: 5.1–5.3).

The Sector Inquiry gave witnesses (and counsel) the chance to be site-specific. It was here that the merits of the various proposals were compared and attempts made by counsel and witnesses to denigrate competing schemes and by local authorities to promote the particular scheme they preferred (if any). Underlying the whole process was the knowledge on everyone's part that only one (if any) of the large retail schemes would be approved by the Secretary of State and that this would be a recommendation of the Inspector. We have noted that two of the large schemes lay in the Borough of Trafford and a third (Barton Locks) just over the border in Salford. The proof of evidence of the Chief Planning Officer of Trafford for the Sector Inquiry was remarkable therefore for the fact that, whilst it commended the advantages of the Trafford Centre, it did so by comparison with the Barton Locks proposal and was silent about the second proposed development in Trafford, at Carrington. The story behind this glaring omission adds little to our analysis of the Trafford Centre and we need not tell it in detail here. However, it is worth a mention because it revolved around the question of inner city impact, or more precisely, impact on urban deprivation. Firstly however, we should note what Mr Stocks thought were the advantages of the Trafford Centre (in itself and by comparison with the Barton Locks Scheme) in terms of its potential impact on the inner cities. Trafford Park (in which the Trafford Centre was to be located), he argued, was as much economically integral to Manchester as it was to Trafford; it had, since its inception, provided employment for people from inner Manchester as well as from Salford and Trafford. In 1981, 40.5 per cent of workers in the Park lived in Trafford and 39.0 per cent in Manchester and Salford (the remainder lived in other parts of, or outside, the Greater Manchester area) (Stocks 1987b: 3.2.2 and Table 3.1: 19). The position of the centre in Trafford Park therefore made it better placed than any of the other schemes on offer (the only reference in the proof that could be taken to include the Carrington Scheme) to serve the needs of the inner cities of the Manchester conurbation. The benefits of increased employment that it would bring would in consequence filter further out into the conurbation's inner cities because its work-force would, if it reflected that of the Park as a whole, come from a draw-area that included more inner city areas (Stocks 1987b: 5.1).

In pressing the advantages of the Trafford Centre (over Barton Locks in particular), Mr Stocks capitalised on its location in Trafford Park (and the Urban Development Corporation), noting that its impact on inner city areas would be all the greater because of its contribution to the regeneration of Trafford Park as a whole (Stocks 1987b: 5.2). What the Trafford Centre had over the other schemes therefore, according to Mr Stocks (its other contributions to the inner cities being common to all the large schemes), was a locational advantage both in terms of its positioning in relation to the conurbation's inner cities and as an integral part of a larger industrial and commercial entity through which its benefits could be projected. And this was the advice he and other senior officers and outside consultants put to Trafford Council before the inquiries. It was advice not taken.

Ironically, the absence of any mention of the Carrington site proposal from the Chief Planning Officer's Sector proof was because this is the scheme that the Borough Planning Committee decided to back – against professional advice.[7] And this it did by (still) playing the 'inner city' card, though in relation to an 'outer city' area. The difference of opinion between members and officers therefore was not one about the potential impact of large retail developments on inner city areas (though the Council as a whole was less enthusiastic about the idea in principle) but rather about *which* 'inner city' areas (or areas of deprivation). The Carrington site lies some one-and-a-half miles from the overspill estate of Partington and is separated from it by the Shell refinery. The estate is relatively isolated, has a low car ownership rate and is relatively poorly served by public transport. It also ranks high among other overspill estates on a number of indicators of deprivation, though not to the same degree as some inner city areas. And it was for the benefits that it might bring to the Partington estate that the Carrington site proposal was promoted by Trafford Council. Of the decision to back Carrington, the Chairman of the Planning Committee had this to say in her proof of evidence to the Sector Inquiry:

> The Secretary of State should know that the decision was actually taken by Council against professional advice.
>
> The Members of Council gave very careful thought to the officers' recommendations and only acted in contravention of what was recognised to be proper professional advice because of the unique (within Trafford) problems of Partington.

(Merry 1987: 2.3)

Then whilst recording the commitment of the Borough Council to the improvement of inner city areas, Ms Merry argued that 'It is. . .the unanimous decision of the Trafford Borough Council, that the inner urban areas are not the only places where severe deprivation and social problems can be found' (Merry 1987: 2.3). And:

> It is absolutely central to the Council's approach to the Carrington application that it provides the potential for providing employment close to the isolated and economically depressed township of Partington. Indeed, I can say that the determination to take action to meet the needs of this community was the overriding factor affecting the Council decision.

(Merry 1987: 3.1)

Here was the inner city argument stripped down to the very basics. Others may talk of economic regeneration, widening economic bases, local economies and suchlike; the Council saw the matter of a large retail centre in simpler terms: that it would replace jobs lost at the Shell refinery and contribute to efforts to improve Partington.

Trafford Borough Council entered Rule 6 statements in respect both of the Trafford Centre and of the Westside Park Scheme at Carrington (as well as of the smaller schemes at Barton Dock Road). The statement in respect of the Trafford Centre noted that the Council viewed it favourably and rehearsed the various inner city arguments with which we are now familiar (Trafford 1987a: 4), and in particular its role in regenerating Trafford Park (which, it also noted, was a priority policy of the Greater Manchester Structure Plan (Greater Manchester Council 1986: Policy 92)). There were disadvantages attached to the scheme but these were primarily concerned with impact on city centre retailing and traffic generation (Trafford 1987a: 5 and 9). In conclusion, the statement argued, 'The advantages of the Trafford Centre proposal outweigh its disadvantages, *primarily by reason of the benefits it would bring to the residents of the inner city*' (Trafford 1987a: 10, emphasis added).

It is worth recording here therefore that though there were differences within the borough about which scheme to back, no one from the authority, nor any of its expert witnesses, argued against the Trafford Centre or its rival, on grounds of inner city impact. There was unanimity that a large retail centre *could* be beneficial to the inner cities. The opposition on 'inner city' grounds came, as we shall see, from the consortium. How much of this opposition resulted from pique at not being home to one of the large proposals must remain a matter for speculation.

The Trafford Rule 6 Statement on the Trafford Centre viewed it favourably and preferred it (not surprisingly) over the two schemes nearby at Barton Locks but within Salford.[8] It did not however prefer the Trafford Centre to the Carrington scheme; indeed it made no comparisons between the two. Only in the Carrington Rule 6 Statement are the two compared and then only to assert that ' . . .this Council has a preference for Carrington' (Trafford 1987b: 4). This document does not, unlike Merry's evidence, give *primacy* of importance for this preference to the effects on the Partington estate but such arguments feature strongly in it. Partington and neighbouring Carrington, the statement notes, are an Economic and Social 'Priority' Area (the Structure Plan designates them as an Economic and Social *Problem* Area) and as such have a high priority for action. (But so are the inner areas of Manchester and Salford and the inner areas of most older towns in the conurbation as well as seven other overspill estates.) The advantage of the Carrington scheme therefore over all the others would be (so the statement argued) its proximity and benefit to an Economic and Social Problem Area. Why this problem area should take precedence over others is not argued and we must assume that whilst there must be a story there to be told, it is not one that would enlighten our theme. We turn next therefore to look at the evidence brought to the Inquiry by the consortium and the arguments against the 'pure private' strategy. It is worth putting down this marker, however, in conclusion to the views of both Salford and Trafford: that none of the evidence brought by, or on behalf of, these authorities seriously challenged the view that large private sector investment in or near to the inner cities *could* be of benefit to their residents.

We shall look at the evidence of three expert witnesses on behalf of the 'Manchester Consortium' because they raise in one form or another the questions of where investment should be if it is to be of benefit to inner city areas, and of the efficacy of channelling investment into designated areas and discouraging it from going anywhere outside those areas. The position of all seven authorities in the consortium was one of opposition to all the schemes before the inquiries, and this opposition was based largely on the anticipated impact on existing retail centres and, in consequence of this, the potentially adverse impact on inner cities, though the latter was not the main driving force of their opposition.

The inner city issue was dealt with at some length by Roger Tym of Roger Tym and Partners at the Plenary Session.[9] We shall simply note his arguments here (and those of two other expert witnesses) and will reserve a more analytic treatment of them for our evaluation of the private sector strategy in a later chapter. Much of Tym's evidence on inner city impact was given over to describing the contents of the inner area programmes of the Manchester/Salford Partnership and the four programme authorities in Greater Manchester (Bolton, Oldham, Rochdale and Wigan) by way of establishing the nature of the opposition of the seven authorities to large-scale retail investment. The nub of the opposition was that such investment would damage the prospects of regenerating the inner cities and this in turn rested on an indissoluble link between inner cities and city centres. Because this link is vital to the opposition to off-centre retail investment, we shall quote at length from Tym's articulation of it:

> The central question before this Inquiry is whether this present round of applications represents the beginning of a cyclical process that would denude the central business districts of investment confidence which would result in fewer jobs for inner city residents, a material downturn in investment interest in the principal areas of the city and district centres and the eventual collapse of private sector interest in pushing out investment to the inner areas themselves.
>
> (Tym 1987b: 4.5)

And again, he noted the belief of the seven authorities that 'there is a vital link between conserving commercial and investment interest in the retail core and the necessary confidence required to persevere with their inner urban programmes' (Tym 1987b: 4.6).

This link between inner cities and the retail core (the city centres) is established in two ways – through employment and the 'image and confidence necessary for investment *in* the inner areas' (Tym 1987b: 4.6, emphasis added). The employment link is essentially one of job loss and gain in different areas. On the basis of an employment survey carried out by his own firm in 1987, Tym estimated that there were some 5,325 retail workers in Manchester City Centre who lived in the Manchester/Salford designated inner area. He then asserted that

Whilst residents of the inner area depend upon Manchester City Centre retailing alone for approximately 5,325 jobs, any loss of trade from Manchester City to new developments outside the City Centre will cause an equivalent loss of jobs in the city centre.

(Tym 1987b: 4.12)

Setting aside the somewhat tortuous and inaccurate logic involved here, the import of what he is saying seems to be that *if* off-centre developments cause job losses in the city centre, some inner city residents would in all likelihood be among those redundant.

The issues involved really seem to be whether new retail developments off-centre would result in employment losses in the centre, how extensive the latter would be, what the *net* gain/loss would be and whether this would have a differential impact on inner city employees.

The second link between inner cities and city centres is said to be one of image and investment confidence (upon which it appears would depend the confidence of local authorities to press on with their policies of inner city regeneration). Indeed, Tym makes much of the fact that the drafters of various inner area programmes in the conurbation appeared to have put much store by the image of, and confidence in, city centres as a prerequisite to successful inner city regeneration. This being the case, it is clearly an argument to be taken seriously. Let us first survey the issue as it was put by Tym:

Private investment is the litmus test of the success or failure of this Administration's efforts in the inner areas – confidence needs to be created and sustained in the investment climate. Urban Programme authorities stress the importance of maintaining investment confidence as a prerequisite of their success in regenerating their inner areas.

(Tym 1987b: 4.27)

The vitality and viability of inner areas, just as much as town and city centres depends crucially upon sustaining and nurturing an image of success, which itself in turn creates the confidence necessary for more investment and of protection from unwarranted and unjustifiable competition.

(Tym 1987b: 4.29)

An assault upon a town centre is therefore a blow against the inner city; the two are indivisible.

(Tym 1987b: 4.30)

The kernel of the argument is this: that off-centre retail development would damage city centre retailing; the city centre would lose some of its economic buoyancy and become less attractive to new investors; its image as a good place to invest would be compromised, and confidence in its economic vitality would sag. And in some way (unspecified by Tym or those he quotes) this downturn in the fortunes of city centres would undermine the confidence of local authorities rigorously to pursue their inner city policies. The difficulty comes in establishing precisely what the nature of the 'image' link is. That there may be an employment link is clear enough. That a reduced tax-take from a run-down city centre may compromise an authority's ability to provide high standard services for inner city residents is clear enough. And that a run-down and half boarded-up city centre may add to the general air of desuetude over a town is easy to image. But that there is a necessary connection of image and confidence between city centres and inner cities is more difficult to grasp. After all, there is no evidence that thirty years of unprecedented city centre boom between 1960 and the late 1980s did much to halt the unparalleled decline of the inner cities in that same period. The track record of economically buoyant city centres giving the confidence to tackle inner city decay is singularly unimpressive.

The evidence of Professors Robson and Townsend to the Plenary Inquiry on behalf of the consortium was less concerned with the schemes themselves and concentrated to a greater extent on detailing the nature, extent and distribution of deprivation in Greater Manchester. Both proofs of evidence where they were prescriptive argued against more 'outer city' or 'peripheral' development and as such were directed at a debate that was not taking place. We need not dwell on the factual evidence of deprivation that Robson and Townsend brought to the Inquiry because it is undisputed. We shall instead concentrate on the arguments they adduced against any and all of the schemes on offer. Much, it will turn out, hangs upon what constitutes inner and outer cities, city centres and cores and the built-up urban core.

Robson noted that his purpose, having shown the extent of deprivation in the conurbation and demonstrated that inner city polices were beginning to bite, was to

> show that this new process of recovery depends on the core of the conurbation being able to attract future new investment in infrastructure and enterprise which will be put at risk if investment is diverted away from the *built-up urban core*.
>
> (Robson 1987: 1.2, emphasis added)

Elsewhere, whilst making essentially the same point, Robson notes the risk that might be involved if retail investment 'were to be channelled away from *inner areas*', adding this time the danger of alienation among inner city residents (Robson 1987: 6.1, emphasis added). Now presumably, because his case is against all the retail proposals on the table, he counts the Trafford Centre along with the others as being 'away from inner areas'. But if by 'inner areas' he means *designated* inner city policy areas this plainly cannot be true given the centre's location within an urban development corporation. If on the other hand he means spatially distant from inner areas, then a glimpse at Maps 5.1 and 5.2 indicates that this can only be true on a very literal and contained reading of 'inner areas'. The general point that Robson is making is clear enough – and a perfectly valid one – that large-scale investment beyond any spatial reach of the inner areas would be potentially damaging to them if only because of opportunities foregone, and this is just the point he subsequently makes when again referring to the risks involved but this time 'of investment outside the already built-up area and *outside the boundaries of the conurbation*' (Robson 1987: 6.7, emphasis added). But then it is difficult to see what this has to do with investment in a location such as Dumplington or indeed of most of the other proposals before the inquiry.

In drawing his arguments to a close Robson maintains that:

> The critical issue is the balance between the maintenance of a strong regional centre within a revitalised Greater Manchester core and the provision of limited *peripheral investment*. . . .The current proposals tip the balance too strongly in favour of the latter.
>
> (Robson 1987: 7.2, emphasis added)

Our purpose here is not to demonstrate that Robson's arguments are wrong (though as we have shown, they are inconsistent about where the proposed investment was to be) but rather that the idea of the 'inner city' has a tendency to become an *idée fixe*. The fact is of course, as we have argued in Chapter 4, that the inner city cannot be easily or clearly defined other than by arbitrary boundaries (which is the case with those that are designated for special status). Inner cities are characterised by *relative* concentrations of deprivation and what constitutes a concentration depends on where you set the cut-off point on a distribution or, more graphically, how you define the shading bands on a map. It may not matter too much for most purposes (though as we have noted, policies based on area designations do rigidify the whole process), but it does matter when considering the potential impact on areas of deprivation of a major retail investment. Because he did not except it from his arguments, one must suppose that Robson includes the Trafford Centre among investments that are 'away from inner areas', 'outside the already built up area', 'outside the boundaries of the conurbation' and which are 'peripheral'. Others who gave evidence, including most witnesses for Salford and Trafford, and those private sector witnesses who alluded to the inner city question (including one of the present authors), referred to the Trafford Centre as being very much within the precincts of the inner city.

But Robson was not alone in opposing the developments on 'inner city' grounds. Professor Townsend also demonstrated with a wealth of data the extent and distribution of a range of deprivations in the conurbation. In particular, he noted that the concentration of deprivation is only relative, that there are deprived communities scattered throughout the region and that numerically, more deprived people live outside the inner cities (however defined) than within them (Townsend 1987: 7.1, 7.2). However, the substance of his submission was that 'Since *outer city developments* favour the affluent parts of the conurbation at the expense of the poorer inner areas. . .they deserve to be better controlled to the benefit of society', and

> where a choice exists, investment should be directed to those areas where social problems are greatest, in order to redress some of the balance of lost investment, lack of job opportunity and restricted economic activity.
>
> (Townsend 1987: 19.9, emphasis added, 19.10)

Again, there seems to be a mythologising of the inner city. The Trafford Centre, along with the other developments, is consigned to the 'outer city' and as such will damage inner areas, will not redress the balance of lost investment and so on. But is this not guilt by association? Can the potential benefit to the inner areas of a Trafford Centre be so cavalierly dismissed just by calling it an 'outer city development'? The question that all this raises is *where* does £150 million worth of development providing 6,500 jobs have to be located if it is to be of benefit to the inner city if Dumplington (see Map 5.1) is in the 'outer city'?

LOCATION

We have seen in the previous section that in debate about the desirability or otherwise of the Trafford Centre, and its potential impact for good or ill on the inner cities, much turns on its location in respect of designated areas, areas of deprivation, the inner areas and so on. It might be thought that the location of a 304-acre site was fairly indisputable, but for the purposes of inner city impact this is apparently not the case. We should not of course be surprised that the ideas of 'inner' and 'outer' city are spatially flexible (we have said as much) but both reification of a discrete inner city and the designation of areas with defined boundaries tend to rigidify the concepts. In this brief section we wish to place the Trafford Centre in its spatial relationship to various designated areas and to the main relative concentrations of selected components of deprivation in the Manchester conurbation.

The latter tend to be, as we have noted, artefacts of the way in which we manipulate our statistics which is why we use the term 'relative concentrations' and why we shall not be too dogmatic about where the boundaries of such concentrations lie.

The purpose of identifying the proximity of the Trafford Centre to special status areas and areas of deprivation is not to attribute to the centre any special importance in itself but rather because a scheme of this size with a job-generating capacity in excess of 6,000 cannot locate in the city centre and probably not in the inner city either (even if it were desirable, which we shall argue it is not). At issue then is whether it could be of benefit to inner cities where it could locate – in Dumplington. And this is just one example of a more general case – whether such large-scale developments can be of benefit (at least so far as proximity is concerned) to inner city areas when located in the only places where they *can* locate. But of course, if the argument that, to be of benefit to the inner city, investment must be located *in* it is rigidly adhered to, then the answer is a foregone conclusion. It is not an argument we wish rigidly to adhere to.

The location of the Trafford Centre site in relation to a number of components of deprivation is shown in Maps 8.1 to 8.5. The extent to which relative concentrations of these deprivations fall within a five-mile radius of the Trafford Centre site varies (as does their overall distribution), but with the exception of 'youth unemployment' (see Map 8.3) and taking account of outlying concentrations, it does appear to be the *bulk* of the spatial concentration in each case. It may of course be argued that five miles does not represent close proximity when we are talking about journey-to-work distances (and time, and cost) which, given our analysis of the nature of the penetrative effects of new investment on urban deprivation, are the determining components of spatial relationships. This is almost certainly true for the majority of unskilled and semi-skilled workers at present and if we accept that such workers will never travel this sort of distance to work, then it must follow that their future employment needs will depend on job growth in the inner areas (if that is where they live). But then we are effectively ruling out any large-scale job-generating scheme (or, if large enough sites were available in the inner cities we will be accepting the close intermixing of residential with commercial, retail and manufacturing uses). However, this does seem to be an unnecessarily limiting constraint to accept when planning for long-term job growth. And because the average journey-to-work distance for unskilled and semi-skilled workers is *now* considerably less than five miles, it does not mean that it always will be, given the range of possibilities for subsidised (and frequent) public and privately provided mass transport. We shall return to the question of accessibility later in this chapter.

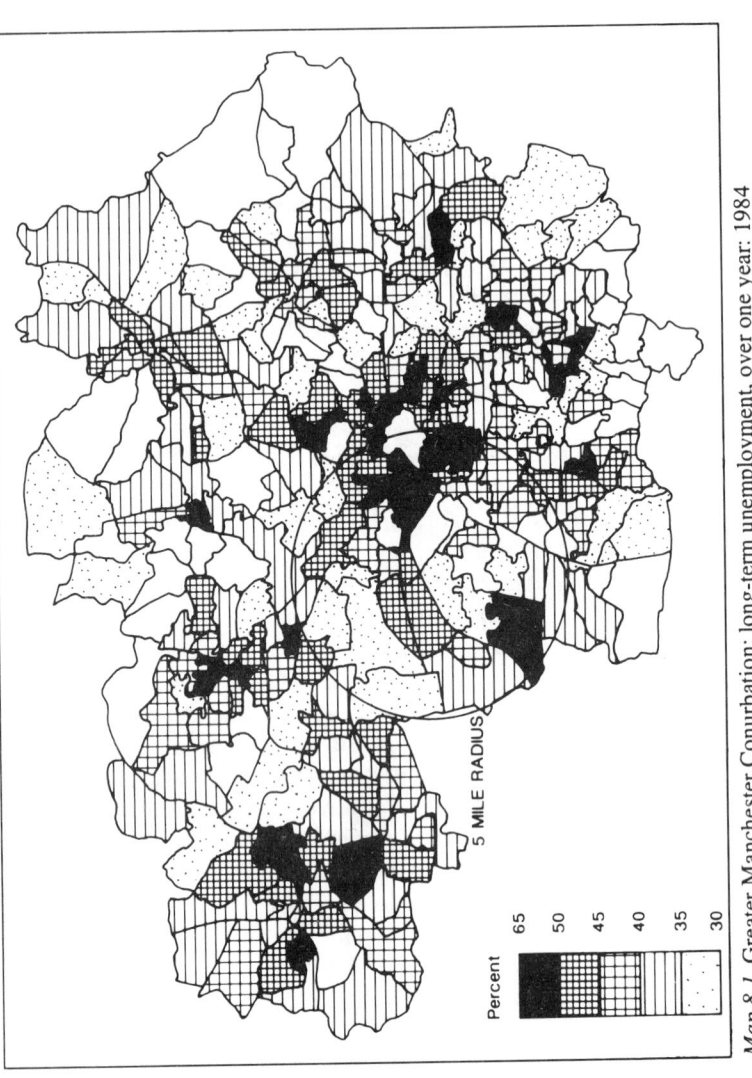

Map 8.1 Greater Manchester Conurbation: long-term unemployment, over one year: 1984

Percent

65
50
45
40
35
30

5 MILE RADIUS

Whatever the particular arguments about feasible travel-to-work distances, it is clear from these maps that the site of the Trafford Centre can in no way be said to be divorced from the main loci of relative concentrations of (at least some) deprivations. Whatever its impact would have been on the inner areas, for good or bad, it would not have been the same as it would have been had it been peripherally located (as some witnesses seem to have been arguing at the inquiries). Furthermore, we have seen that the site of the Trafford Centre is within the designated area of the Trafford Park Development Corporation. To argue therefore that investment on that site might not be of benefit to the inner areas, and indeed, might be harmful to them, appears to confound both the entire strategy of the development corporation and the plausibility of its location.

The location of the Trafford Centre in relation to relative concentrations of unemployment is further demonstrated by Table 8.2, which lists the fifteen wards (1981 boundaries) in Manchester, Salford and Trafford with the highest 1987 unemployment rates (male and female) in rank order and an estimate of what proportion, spatially, of each ward falls within a five-mile radius.

Table 8.2   Wards with high unemployment: Manchester, Salford and Trafford: 1987

Ward	*% Unemployed*	*Proportion in 5-mile radius*
Hulme (M)	46.2	All
Moss Side (M)	33.9	7/8
Cheetham (M)	31.5	¼
Ardwick (M)	30.9	–
Collegiate Church (M)	30.2	2/3
Albert Park (S)	29.7	All
Miles Platting (M)	28.1	–
St Pauls and Docks (S)	27.8	All
Alexandra (M)	27.0	All
St Mathias, Trinity and Crescent (S)	26.9	All
Clifford (T)	26.8	All
Longsight (M)	26.7	–
Langworth and Seedley (S)	25.8	All
Mandley Park (S)	25.8	½
Beswick (M)	25.7	–

Sources: Census Digests 1981, Manchester, Salford, Trafford
Data: Planning Departments, Manchester, Salford, Trafford, 1987

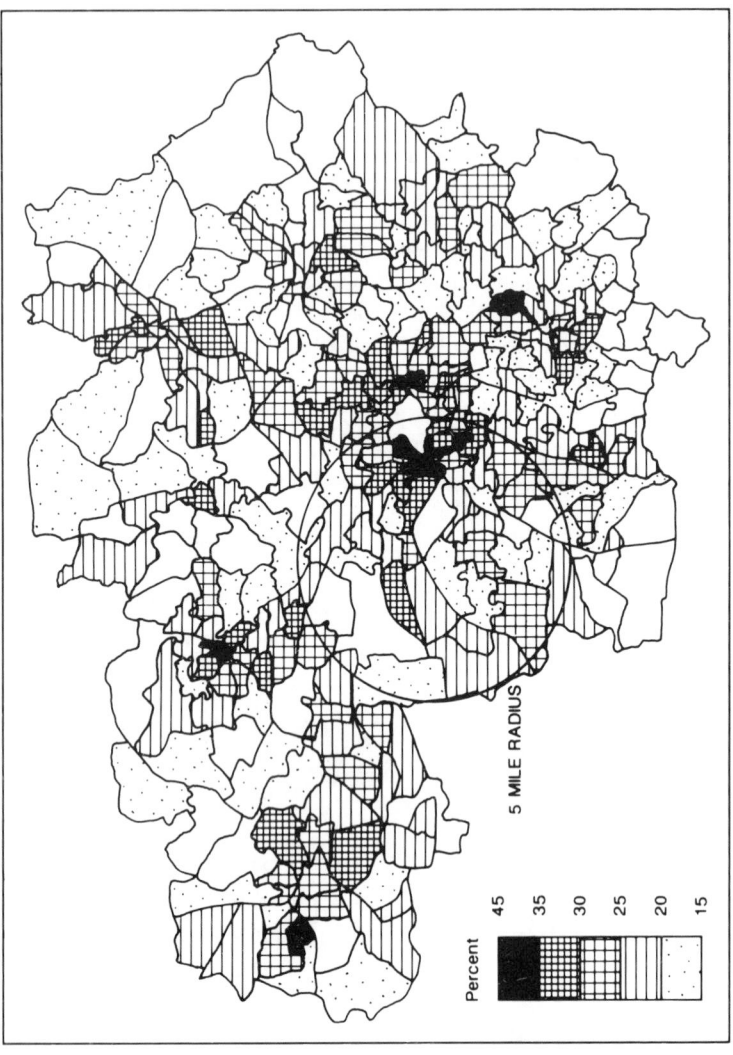

Percent	
45	(solid black)
35	(cross-hatch)
30	(dense grid)
25	(vertical lines)
20	(light vertical)
15	(stipple)

5 MILE RADIUS

Map 8.2 Greater Manchester Conurbation: long-term unemployment, over two years

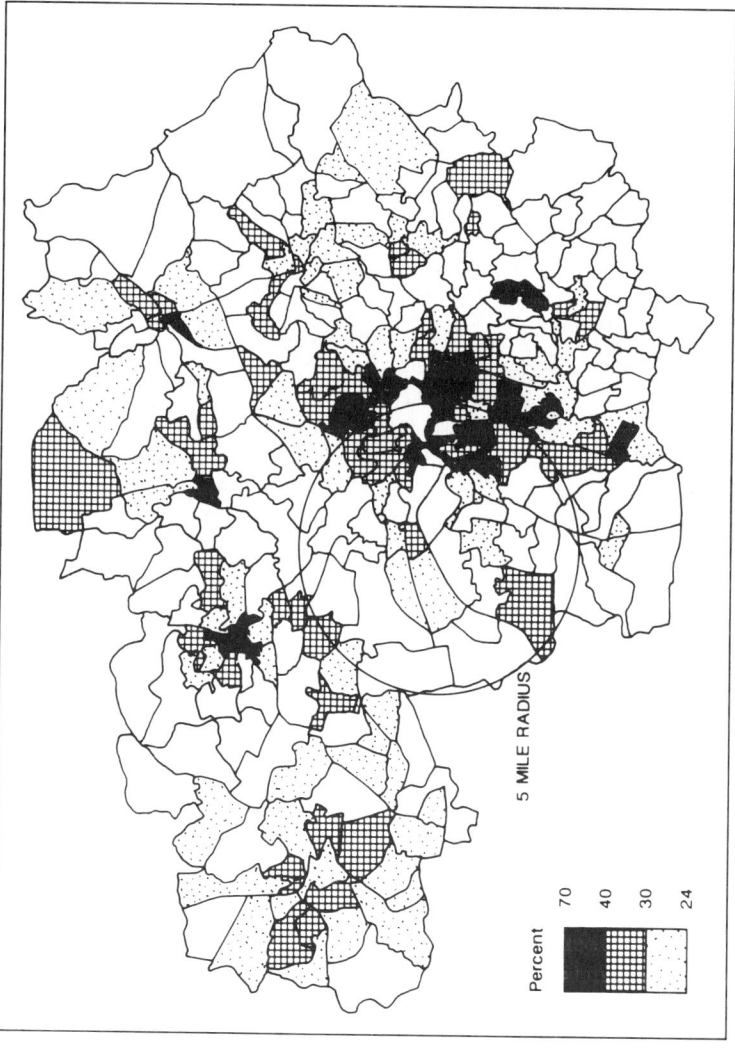

Percent

70
40
30
24

5 MILE RADIUS

Map 8.3 Greater Manchester Conurbation: youth unemployment: 1984

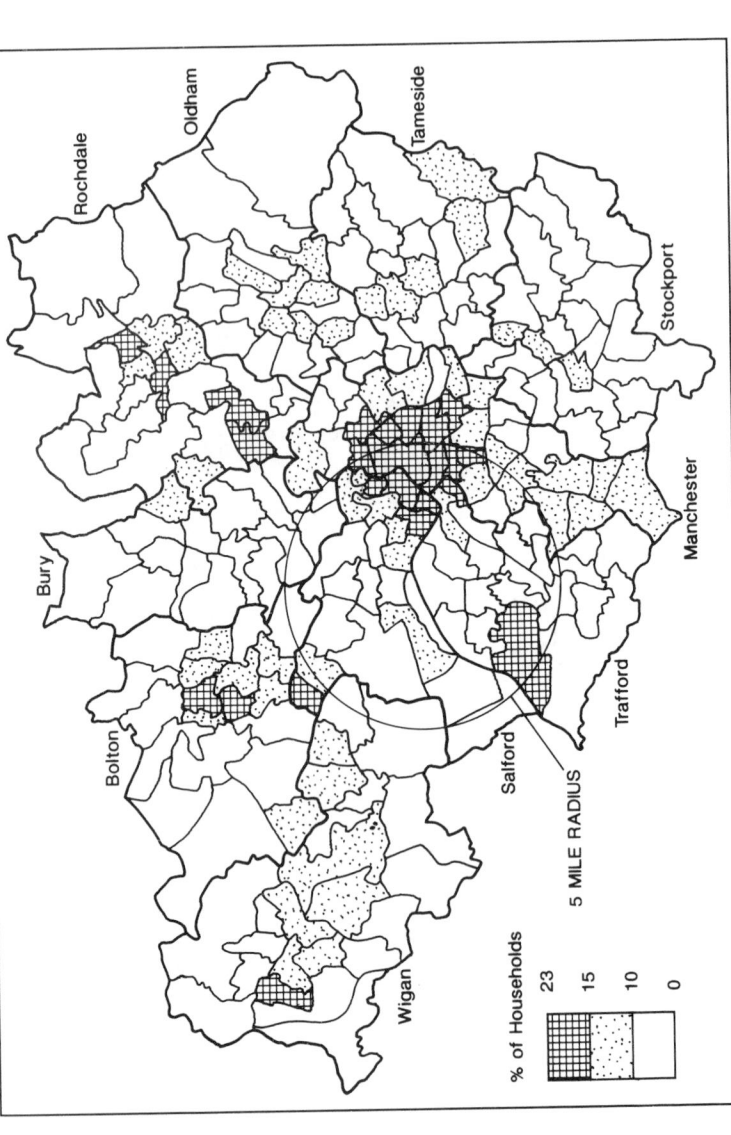

Map 8.4 Greater Manchester Conurbation: households with head unemployed or sick as a percentage of all households, by ward: 1981

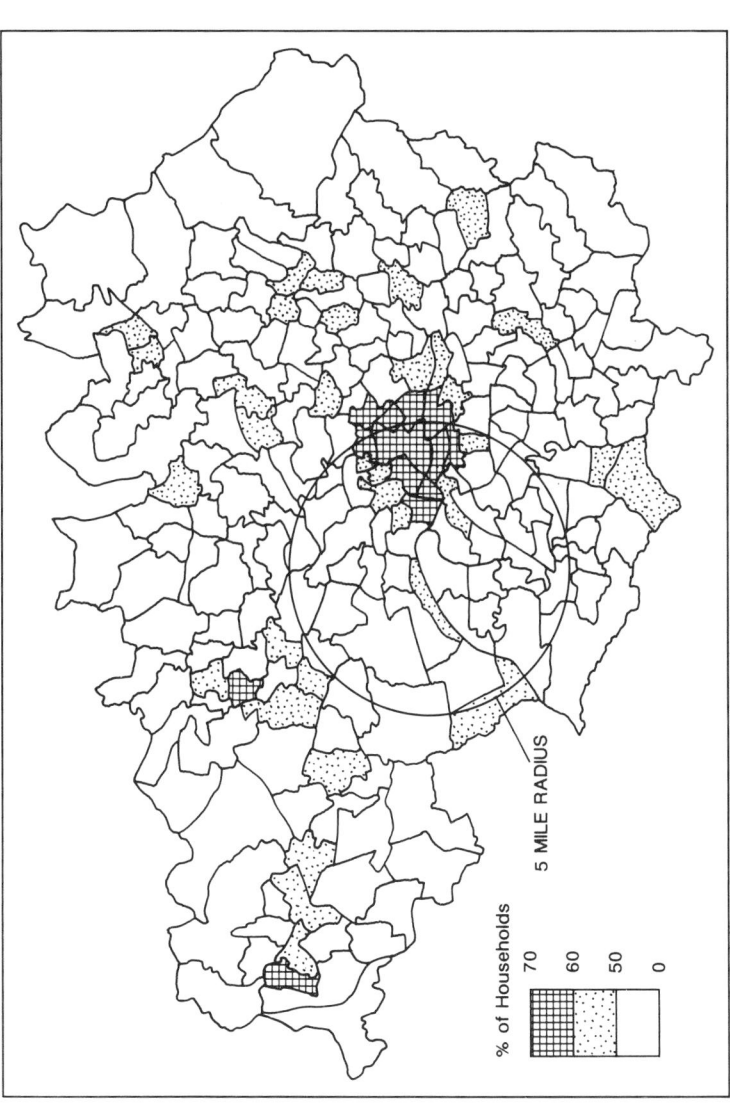

% of Households

70
60
50
0

5 MILE RADIUS

Map 8.5 Greater Manchester Conurbation: low-income households (households with head in semi- or unskilled occupation as a percentage of all households) by ward: 1981

It is possible, using these and supplementary data, to produce a rough estimate of the numbers of unemployed claimants living within the five-mile radius of the Trafford Centre site. Using percentage unemployment rates and numbers in the labour force for each ward and apportioning these by the amount of each ward that lies within the radius provides us with (an admittedly approximate) figure of 35,000. Seven of the fifteen wards fall wholly within five miles of the centre plus some seven-eighths of Moss Side, two-thirds of Collegiate Church, one-half of Mandley Park, a quarter of Cheetham, and nothing of the remaining four.

There are other locational factors that are of relevance to the potential impact of a development such as the Trafford Centre. We have already noted that as well as being located in the development corporation area, it also falls in an area designated in the Greater Manchester Structure Plan as an 'Economic and Social Problem' Area. Policy 92 of the Structure Plan states that 'In putting into effect the policies and general proposals of the plan, regard will be had to [their] economic and social needs' (Greater Manchester Council 1986: Policy 92; see also Greater Manchester Council Planning Department 1983).

Finally, the Trafford Centre site lies only a mile from the boundary of the Manchester/Salford Partnership area and a five-mile radius takes in more than one half of this area which includes the centre of Manchester and the 'core' inner areas of the conurbation. This is the area in which Manchester and Salford have decided to concentrate their urban pro-gramme resources and we may reasonably assume it to be *the* priority area for inner city policy purposes. Once again, the tyranny of area designations has a tendency (exacerbated by the fact that there really are boundaries drawn on a map) to view all action (including private investment (Manchester/Salford Partnership 1985/6, para 3.1)) within the designated area as beneficial and anything outwith it as potentially harmful. There is no site large enough and acceptable to developers within the Partnership area for a scheme the size of the Trafford Centre. It must be outside. Does this mean that it would be potentially harmful? Clearly, it is schemes like the Trafford Centre that test the logic of area designations. We should add however that this does not mean that such schemes will not be harmful – the balance of possibilities has yet to be established – but rather that it is prematurely to foreclose argument to say that they might be harmful *because* they are not in designated areas.

The question of proximity to areas of residential concentration of the deprived, including the unemployed, resolves itself, so far as the impact of new investment on deprivation is concerned, not entirely, but mainly, into one of accessibility for employment purposes. (This at least is the logical consequence of our analysis of the logic of economic regeneration. But even if a greater prominence were given to the idea of an 'inner city economy' than we are inclined to provide, employment proximity would still loom large in the analysis.) Our evaluation of the potential impact of the Trafford Centre (which forms part of the substance of Chapter 9) will therefore require us to say more about the accessibility of the site than we have so far.

For the purposes of establishing the proximity of the Trafford Centre site to areas of relative concentration of deprivation we have used a five-mile radius. Whilst acknowledging that this is probably more than the average journey-to-work distance for unskilled and semi-skilled workers, it has been argued that it is not an unreasonable distance given a longer-term perspective (and the hope, if a regeneration strategy worked, that skill levels – and with them, income – would be raised).

Proximity is not the same as accessibility however, especially for journeys by public transport. It so happens that Trafford Park as a whole is poorly served by public transport particularly at off-peak periods from the inner areas of Manchester and Salford, and, to a lesser extent, Trafford (Stocks 1987b: 5.9). But that provides no reason for assuming that that must always be the case. Even so, 23 per cent of all journeys to work in Trafford Park originate in the inner areas of Manchester, Trafford and Salford, and of those 35 per cent are by public transport. For Manchester alone, 50 per cent of work journeys to Trafford Park originating in the inner city are by public transport. Furthermore, proximity cannot be altered but accessibility can. The Trafford Park Investment Strategy, the principles of which were subsequently adopted by the Development Corporation, includes detailed proposals for improved public transport provision concomitant with projected employment growth (Trafford Park Investment Strategy 1986: 2.3, 6.3).

The location of the Trafford Centre in relation to relative concentrations of deprivation is therefore at the crux of much of the debate (at least as it was conducted at the public inquiries) about its impact on the inner cities of the Manchester Conurbation. In our brief review of its locational characteristics here, we have sought not to place undue weight on its position within the development corporation area. This we have done because we shall subsequently wish to evaluate the potential impact that the Trafford Centre might have had independently of its role in the development corporation strategy. It is no part of our argument therefore that being a part of the development corporation would automatically have made it beneficial to inner areas either locationally or strategically.

PROJECTED JOB CREATION

The main direct impact that a development like the Trafford Centre would have on urban deprivation is, as we have seen, through the net new jobs it created that could and would be taken by previously unemployed inner city residents. There are two quite separate components to this process. The first concerns the number and types of job created; the second, measures that might be taken to maximise the chances of unemployed inner city residents getting them. Anticipated job creation is discussed in this section. Ways of maximising take up by inner city residents we shall discuss when we come to evaluate the enterprise strategy in Chapter 9.

It was estimated at the time of the inquiries that the retail component of the Trafford Centre would create approximately 5,000 jobs of which, based on analyses of the Metro Centre in Gateshead, some 45 per cent would be full-time and 55 per cent part-time. Also using the Metro Centre as a model, it was estimated that 21 per cent of these jobs might be taken by males and 79 per cent by females, though the sex distribution would be subject to more uncertainties (Stocks 1987b: 5.3). In addition, the leisure complex was expected to create some 1,500 jobs in all with a somewhat higher proportion of full-time jobs than in the retail centre (Tibbott 1987: 18). If this employment growth were to be the effective agent in the process of ameliorating deprivation, it matters a great deal what kinds of job are involved. To be available to those who need them, they would have to be at such skill levels as would match those of the unemployed or to which they could be trained. Once more, using the model of the Metro Centre, the figures in Table 8.3 give the approximate distribution over job types and levels.

No comparable data were available for the leisure complex but it is likely that this would have broadened and shifted the distribution because of the wider range of jobs it would have provided. If we confine our remarks to the retail centre, however, and if we make the not unreasonable assumption that maximum impact on deprivation would result from the currently unemployed with least prospects (say the unskilled and semi-skilled) gaining employment, then we can see that given requisite (and realistic) levels of job training, all but the 20 per cent of management jobs would be available to this group. There is of course a reservation, but

Table 8.3 Trafford Centre: job generation by type

	%		%
Management	20	Stock handling	3
Sales	60	Security	2
Clerical	7	Cleaning	2
Catering	5		

Source: Stocks 1987b: Table 5.1b

unfortunately not one we can quantify. The approximate job creation of 6,500 is a gross figure. The development of a scheme such as the retail component of the Trafford Centre might lead to some retail closures in the city centre (and possibly in inner city areas). Jobs would be lost in consequence and the net gain would be less than 6,500. (However, it is worth comparing this approximate figure of 6,500 with the 10,500 permanent and 2,500 temporary jobs created by *all* twenty-four enterprise zones in Great Britain combined, since their inception in 1981/82 (National Audit Office 1990: 4.25).) Furthermore, in addition to jobs in the centre, the construction of the site itself would have created an estimated 2,000 new jobs over a period of two-and-a-half years and, though not permanent, these could have contributed in the short term at least to a reduction in unemployment.

What these figures give us therefore is an indication of the magnitude of job creation by a scheme such as the Trafford Centre. These are jobs that could be available to inner city residents under certain conditions. If events so conspired that very few of the new jobs went to previously unemployed people in areas of deprivation, then by our own analysis of the process by which enterprise could benefit inner city residents, the scheme would have failed them. And of course there are many reasons why events might so conspire. What would have to be done to minimise the chances of this happening and of maximising the opportunities of inner city residents getting the jobs, is examined subsequently as part of our evaluation. Before leaving the topic of job creation however, we should say a word about costs.

Creating jobs can be a costly business. The Trafford Park Investment Strategy estimated that the net public expenditure per gross additional job in retailing in Trafford Park would be of the order of £3,900. The Manchester Ship Canal Company proposed the Trafford Centre Scheme independently of the development strategy and without benefit of any public subsidy. The net cost to public funds therefore of jobs created in the centre would have been negligible and probably zero. These figures can be compared with the estimates in the Regional Industrial Development White Paper of 1983 that the cost per additional job created in the assisted areas in the 1970s was approximately £35,000 at 1982 prices (House of Commons 1983) and the estimates prepared for the Department of the Environment of the cost per additional job created in the enterprise zones, which produced an average figure of £30,000 and a ceiling of £48,000 (National Audit Office 1990: 4.25-4.26).

THE SEQUEL: RECOMMENDATIONS AND DECISION

Our interest has focused on the Trafford Centre as an example of 'pure private' investment that would have had an impact on inner city areas. The fact that it was subject to a local inquiry is of interest largely in so far as the inquiry generated a large volume of data and argument that are of value to our evaluation of the likely impact that the centre may have had. Never the less, the sequel to the inquiry is worth telling if only briefly, because once again, the inner city issue featured strongly in the inspectors' recommend-ations and in the Secretary of State's decision (or rather, non-decision).

In summary, the Report of the Plenary Session argued that one, and only one, large retail centre could be justified and that none of the three largest proposals, if they went ahead, would damage the inner areas of the conurbation. The Report of the Sector Session recommended that outline planning permission be granted to the Trafford Centre and that its location would bring undoubted benefits for the inner areas. It was recommended that all other applications be refused. The Secretary of State agreed with the Inspectors' recommendation in respect of the Trafford Centre (but not the others) except on one point relating to traffic generation on the M63 motorway, but in the light of post-inquiry evidence from the Department of Transport declined to determine the application and referred the matter back to the Manchester Ship Canal Company.

That section of the Inspector's report on the Plenary Session dealing with inner city matters was lifted almost *en bloc* from the proof of evidence presented at the inquiry by one of the present authors (see Edwards 1987a). And since we have already noted that the recommendation was that the Trafford Centre (and only the Trafford Centre) be granted outline per-mission, it will be apparent that this evidence was supportive of it (in so far as the inner city impact was concerned). But having declared – not so much an interest in as a view on – the desirability of the Trafford Centre (but again, only from the inner city viewpoint), it must be said that this does not necessarily extend to a more general case about the effectiveness of the enterprise strategy writ large. On that we shall remain agnostic until we have completed our evaluation. And as we shall see subsequently, what might have seemed a good idea in 1987 may look decidedly less attractive in 1992.

The gist of the Inspectors' remarks on the three main retail proposals in relation to inner city impact may be summarised by quoting a few selected passages:

Any development which provides jobs, and stimulates investment near to those [economic and social problem] areas is beneficial.

In the case of the three main proposals. . . . very little or possibly no public investment would be required. Surely such an opportunity cannot be turned down.

Rather than undermining urban policy initiatives, alternative shopping facilities. . .will provide jobs for those in the problem areas.

The choice is not whether this development should occur in one of the locations selected by developers or in Central Manchester. The choice is whether the investment should be allowed where it is proposed or whether it should take place at all. Certainly, Professors Robson and Townsend put forward no material to support the proposition that allowing any of the major schemes would involve the diversion of funds from, or the discouragement of, investment in the inner city.

The major schemes would have no adverse effect on the social and economic problems of the inner city, indeed they would bring substantial benefits to those areas.

(All quotations from Department of the Environment 1989c: 7.4.14; 7.4.17; 7.4.22; 7.4.27; 7.4.28)

The report of the Sector Inquiry, including the Inspectors' recommendations to the Secretary of State in respect of each application, came down firmly in favour of the Trafford Centre. Two brief quotations will suffice to give the essence of the Inspectors' remarks so far as inner city matters were concerned:

Large scale new development would inevitably create environmental problems within the inner city, the ideal location would therefore be on the edge of the inner city but with good access for inner city residents. The Trafford Centre met these criteria.

Development in the inner city which did not have damaging effects on the environment would be desirable and would help regeneration. Such development was, however, unlikely to include large scale shopping; the construction of the Trafford Centre on the edge of the inner city would therefore not delay redevelopment in the inner city.

(Quotations from Department of the Environment 1989d: 4.2.3; 4.2.10)

It is worth noting then that in giving the Trafford Centre the green light, the inspectors had lent some weight to the probability of large-scale development causing environmental problems were it to be located (even if it could be located) *in* the inner cities. This is taken to be a reference to the undesirability of mixed and incompatible land use and must be seen as inconsistent with any assertion that for development to be of benefit to the inner cities, it must be located in them.

The Secretary of State's letter of response was issued at the same time as the Plenary and Sector reports were released. The letter had this to say about the Trafford Centre: 'With regard to the proposed Trafford Centre, the Secretary of State agrees with the Inspector's conclusions except for. . . .' (Department of the Environment 1989e: para 8). (The remainder of this paragraph and the substance of the decision not to permit the Trafford Centre then concerns issues of traffic flow on the M63 motorway which was the reason for non-determination.) It must be assumed therefore that the Secretary of State agreed with the substance of the Inspectors' recommendations in respect of inner city impact and with their arguments concerning the undesirability of large-scale job creation developments taking place *in* the inner city.

The Secretary of State declined to determine the applications before him,[10] including the Trafford Centre, though this was his preferred option. The reason for the non-determination was largely the result of a post-inquiry objection by the Department of Transport based upon its own traffic-generation estimates which suggested that additional (fourth) lanes would be required on the M63 northbound between junctions 2 and 3 and southbound between junctions 3 and 4. (These estimates were subsequently to be revised.) The stage was then set for another round of negotiations between the Ship Canal Company and the Department of Transport but the ground rules were clear: the company would have to acquire the land and pay for the construction of the two new lanes. The Secretary of State's letter invited further representations, none of which in the event materially altered the situation that, subject to traffic objections, Trafford Centre was still the preferred option. A response to these representations (including one of considerable significance from the Department of Transport) was issued by the DoE on 7 May 1991 which again invited further response within twenty-one days.

Meanwhile, the Trafford Centre was being drawn on to an increasingly complex checkerboard involving new players with a strong interest in the game. At the time of the original inquiry and its immediate aftermath, the development corporation was in its nascent stage (and submitted only a brief letter to the inquiry expressing its preferred use for the Dumplington site). In the intervening years however the corporation has of necessity developed a stronger interest in the future of the Trafford Centre and this has become inextricably linked to whether and how the Greater Manchester Passenger Transport Executive proceeds with the LRT line (see Chapter 5).

The Secretary of State's letter of 7 May 1991 noted in respect of new evidence that the Department of Transport, on the basis of 'more reliable assumptions', no longer thought that a fourth southbound lane on the M63 was required and so this (post-inquiry) objection fell. The fourth north-bound lane and sundry other improvements were however still necessary. The immediate response of the Development Corporation to this letter was to call for early talks between the Ship Canal Company, the Department of Transport and itself to agree necessary road alterations and to reach a legal agreement on them. The corporation went further however in a subsequent and more detailed submission (Trafford Park Development Corporation 1991c) which noted the new developments and a proposal by the Department of Transport that the Ship Canal Company enter an agreement under Section 278 of the Highways Act 1980 with the department to carry out the necessary works at the company's cost. It then went on to give support for the need for the Department of Transport to secure the necessary improvements to the M63 and noted that the Ship Canal Company was prepared to enter such an agreement and bear any costs that might be considered reasonable in consequence of the Trafford Centre Development. It therefore urged that the talks referred to in its shorter submission be held immediately.

However, as we saw above, the future of the Trafford Centre is now bound up with the future of the Light Rapid Transit System and that brings another actor – the Passenger Transport Executive (PTE) – into the game. The PTE wants to develop the light railway into the Park but cannot pay for it; the money must come from the private sector. The Ship Canal Company wants it because it will (if it does not stop short in the centre of the Park) provide a direct passenger link from the centre of Manchester to the Trafford Centre. And the Development Corporation wants it for the image and kudos it will bring to the UDA. The question is – as ever – who is going to pay and how much?

In August 1989, the Department of Transport, in outlining the 'unacceptable' transportation implications of the Trafford Centre, noted the (then) absence of firm support for the LRT being extended into Trafford Park as a supplementary factor to the motorway difficulties. For the department therefore, the LRT is an important (and possibly a necessary) component of the future of the Trafford Centre. The development corporation has hitched its response to this contingency, arguing that it believes that 'the provision of L.R.T. through Trafford Park to the Trafford Centre is both feasible and desirable' (Trafford Park Development Corporation 1991c, para 4.2). It then goes on to express the wish that the Ship Canal Company and the Greater Manchester Passenger Transport Executive would meet to reach agreement on terms and provide a continuing commitment to the LRT.

In interpreting these events, it is probably true to say that the development corporation wants (and possibly needs) the LRT more than does the Ship Canal Company. It would certainly be an image booster. But it is easier for the corporation to urge commitment and action on the part of others because it will not pick up the bill at the end. The Ship Canal Company meanwhile faces a changed retailing climate in which the financial prospects of a Trafford Centre look less attractive than they did five years ago. This may only be a 'blip' in long-term upward trends but it is not the most auspicious moment to 'buy' permission for the Trafford Centre not only with a new motorway lane but a new LRT as well. But the development corporation needs the Trafford Centre as well as the LRT. It is a large site (60 per cent of the remaining developable land in the UDA) and its use has been blighted for four years by planning indecision. There is no doubt a great deal of hard bargaining to come.

Now all of this may seem to have little to do with the problem of the inner cities. But if we suppose (to presume for a moment on the content of a later chapter) that the Trafford Centre would have been of benefit to inner city areas in some way or other, then the relevance of the closing chapters of the story is just that *it is not yet there*. And it isn't there for a variety of reasons, some of which may be predictable (such as a ponderous planning process) but others (like economic recession) are predictable only by pundits in hindsight. It is one thing for a development to be subject to the vagaries of the economic climate so far as the developer (and potential shoppers) are concerned; it is quite another matter if it is to be used as an instrument of social policy. It means, in short, that social policy becomes subject to the same climatic uncertainties. The message *might* of course be 'don't rely on private enterprise for incidental social spin-offs'. But if this is true of a Trafford Centre, is it any less true of publicly subsidised levered development?

NOTES

1   Details of the various applications are given in the Trafford Park Rule 6 Statement (Trafford Centre), Town and Country Planning Act 1971 Section 35, Town and Country Planning (Inquiries Procedure) Rules 1974 (Trafford 1987a: 1).

2   Brent Cross in London has some 79,000 square feet of retail floorspace, and the Metro Centre in Gateshead some 1.5m square feet.

3   Details of the various schemes are given in the Inspectors' Reports on the Plenary and Sector Inquiries: Department of the Environment 1989c; 1989d.

4   There was a general preference for 'high-technology' use but, given the amount of unused land in Trafford Park, designating particular plots for particular use was not driven by strict exigencies. Certainly there are no inherent features to Dumplington that make it especially suitable for high-technology use (see Stocks 1987b: 68–9; Salford City Council 1987b: 9).

5   Nor shall we concern ourselves with the attempts by witnesses for the Trafford Centre to do the same of rival schemes.

6   We shall have more to say about centre city investment as against inner city investment later in this chapter. Confusion of the two allowed a great deal of obfuscation in some evidence put to the inquiries.

7   But not to the exclusion of 'supporting' the Trafford Centre.

8 There was a second smaller proposal at Barton Locks as well as the one we have already mentioned.

9 Roger Tym and Partners was one of the five firms which drew up the Trafford Park Investment Strategy.

10 Except the Carrington Scheme which was refused planning permission.

9   The reach of private enterprise

At a superficial level, the enterprise solution to the problems of the inner cities has an appealing simplicity. Once the root cause of these problems has been traced back to a degenerated economic infrastructure, logic dictates that regeneration is the answer and since this means, at its most basic, both wealth and job creation, then the most effective – indeed the *only* – instrument to bring it about is private enterprise. And the only role that governments need play is to help private enterprise choose the appropriate locations, which in effect means tipping the economic balance in favour of inner city locations in the competition to attract investment. After all, companies can hardly be expected to bear the economic costs of locating in a less favourable area just because there might be social benefits attached to their doing so. At its simplest therefore, and leaving aside for the moment the paraphernalia of partnership and 'single-minded bodies', the enterprise solution to urban deprivation is really a reverse replay of thirty years of industrial location policy (see Goddard and Champion 1983; Cullingworth 1985; Balchin and Bull 1987).

At an equally simplistic level, it seems obvious that the strategy won't work, and incredible that anyone should ever have thought that it would. Think of that young man in the LDDC advertisement doing deals on his mobilephone while windsurfing through the foam of St Katherine's Dock. Is he the same man from the council estate in Tower Hamlets who last week was queuing for his dole? (Has he also bought his council flat? And taken out BUPA insurance? All the hallmarks of enterprise man. He will need the BUPA insurance if he gets Weil's disease from swallowing too much Thames water.) All is not what it seems in Docklands and this is particularly so for those who were the intended beneficiaries. How much of it has been fantasy? And to what extent have the 'single-minded bodies' (and their local populations) been the victims of their own glossy hype? As ever, the answer depends on the perceived purposes. There is no doubt that at one level, at least some of the examples we have examined have been successful. Fit and proper homes and environments (well, apart from the water) will have been created for enterprise man and woman. But this is (or was intended to be) inner city policy and the ultimate beneficiaries were going to be the urban deprived, either by way of spin-off from the regeneration process or because they too would be transformed into enterprise people. So far as this evaluation of the enterprise approach is concerned therefore, the high-gloss output of the agencies we have looked at – the square metreage of office space created, kilometres of road laid, gearing ratios, etc. – are means to an end: they are not in themselves indicators of success.

We have outlined the ground rules for our evaluation of the 'enterprise solution' in earlier chapters. We need only enter a brief reminder here about the problems that make up urban deprivation and about the aims and (intuited) logic of the enterprise strategy. That done, we shall use the evidence from our four case-studies to give substance to the evaluation of a number of components of the strategy, as one for dealing with urban deprivation.

THE PROBLEMS

In Chapter 3, we itemised the components of what has generically become known as 'urban deprivation' and then grouped them into six categories. The 'logic' of the economic regeneration strategy was then applied to each in order to establish at least the potential of such a strategy for reaching into deprivation. It is this potential reach of enterprise that we test in this chapter against the evidence from the case studies.

Briefly to recapitulate our earlier analysis therefore, the six types of deprivation and their susceptibility to the impact of economic regeneration were as follows:

characteristics of people and households, some of which might be directly affected (such as unemployment) and others of which might benefit from a trickle effect;

environmental factors which might be directly improved though the emphasis is more likely to be on investment-attracting environmental works rather than domestic-scale improvement that might be of more direct benefit to local people;

housing factors, the improvement of which was identified as not being a direct component of the enterprise strategy, though housing provision may be made by some agencies either for general purposes or as a peripheral investment inducement;

education factors, which again, apart from the (very important) training

component, do not form part of the regeneration strategy;
service provision, which whilst not a direct part of the regeneration strategy might be affected by it if only indirectly as a result of the enhanced image of the area (so far as financial services are concerned) or as a result of enhanced resources from a strengthened tax-base;
economic and financial factors, which will, rightly speaking, be the immediate target for a regeneration strategy but the improvement of which will only be a means to the reduction of other, and in particular personal and household, deprivations.

Given this analysis of urban deprivation therefore, and using it as a specification of the problems, some of which it is the purpose of the enterprise strategy to relieve, we can see that (as we have noted before) the logic of the regeneration strategy must be such as to impact mainly on the first of these categories either directly, through employment generation or through the trickle effect. (The direct impact on the last category will, as we point out above, be a means to this end.)

The focus of our evaluation therefore is on the deprivation-related impact of the enterprise strategy itself. This is not to say however that some of the agencies we have examined will not, in varying degrees, make a more direct impact on some aspects of deprivation by way of housing, environmental and particularly social provisions. These would of course constitute a part of the evaluation of the overall impact of our case-study agencies but, in so far as they are not constituents of the enterprise strategy itself, they must remain at the periphery of our focus. It must be noted however, that with the partial exception of Heartlands, the agencies we have examined (and using that term loosely, to include the Trafford Centre) were never intended to be service delivery bodies; their primary, if not sole, purpose was economic regeneration. To the extent that some of them have taken on service delivery functions therefore, they may be tacitly admitting the limitations of the enterprise strategy by itself to effect an acceptable degree of improvement in deprivation.

THE AIMS

The effective evaluation of any policy requires some baseline against which to measure outputs and this will normally take the form of a statement of aims. Without some idea of what the aims of a policy are, and some way of measuring their achievement, then evaluation is denied its basic instruments. It will never be possible to say whether and to what extent a policy has achieved what it set out to do or whether it is worth continuing with or should be altered or replaced.

Unfortunately, as our earlier discussion showed, the aims of recent inner city policies (including the use of urban development corporations) have been couched in only the most general of terms and specifications of success have rarely been more precise than the lifestyle imagery of the glossy brochures. Sadly, not all the elderly, chronically sick and carers of children and elderly parents are going to be able to do their stockbroking whilst windsurfing in St Katherine's Dock. Alas, some may not even achieve it on dry land. But about them, policy is silent.

We know the imagery of success well enough: the cranes on the horizon, the glittering towers, the postmodernist office blocks that adorn the brochures; but it is hard to avoid the conclusion that if this *is* what it is all about, then these policies would work much better if they were nowhere near the inner cities. We have, in consequence of this, adopted the simple expedient of inventing our own aims for the policies of economic regeneration and these have been outlined in Chapter 3. In brief, the enterprise strategy *as inner city policy* can only be deemed to have worked if, as well as, and in consequence of, the glittering towers, there is a reduction in the dependency ratio in the relevant neighbouring areas, reductions in unemployment levels, reductions in the amount of poverty, improvements in the environment, improved services, and (though these are not inherent to the strategy itself) improved housing, health and education provision. But even this, we recognise, is the most bland of statements, devoid as it is (and must be) of any quantification. This, however, takes us to our next topic, but before we move on it is worth emphasising that we are not primarily concerned to evaluate our four case-study institutions as discrete agencies but rather as instruments for the promotion of enterprise. It matters less than it might, therefore, that none of the agencies we examine have overall detailed strategy plans against which to measure their progress. Indeed, it would be impossible to evaluate LDDC, TPDC, or Heartlands against their own strategic aims because they have never been articulated in anything other than very general terms.

INDICATORS

In its 1990 Report on Regenerating the Inner Cities, the National Audit Office argued in respect of Inner Area Programmes that 'Most of the [evaluation] measures so far developed are intermediate measures related to activities rather than effectiveness' (National Audit Office 1990: 3.19). The same criticism can be made of many other inner city strategies, including the urban development corporations.

Typical of the intermediate measures that the NAO was exercised about were such factors as:

numbers of factory units established
numbers of new businesses started up
numbers of jobs created or preserved
numbers of training places established
numbers of visitors/attendances/inquiries (at advice centres, community centres, etc.)
kilometres of waterways/roads improved
hectares of land improved.

They are all by now familiar indicators and if we were to add in the all important 'gearing ratio', they would apply as well to the London Docklands and Trafford Park development corporations, and to Heartlands, as to the inner area programmes. They do not however, as the NAO report implies, measure the extent to which inner cities programmes are reducing urban deprivation. Within the 'logic of the enterprise strategy' as we have outlined it, they are not output measures in themselves but rather the means to other ends. It is, after all, possible to achieve high output on most of these indicators without making any measurable impact on deprivation. The real difficulty therefore lies in devising suitable direct indicators of levels of deprivation in the relevant areas and in being able to apply these over such a period of time during which it would be reasonable to anticipate measurable change, had any occurred. The best sources of data to which to apply these indicators would be either from the censuses or from tailored surveys. The time-span for any significant results to emerge will be somewhat longer than that for which any of our three extant case-studies have been up and running, but as we noted earlier, *some* change ought by now to be evident from the activities of the LDDC and, to a lesser extent, the TPDC. Furthermore, small area data from the 1991 census will be of considerable value for comparison over the first ten years of LDDC.

The particular indicators of 'ultimate' success ought closely to reflect the components of deprivation that we identified in Chapter 3: that is, measures of poverty, unemployment, housing conditions, health, dependency, quality of services and so on. There is by now an extensive literature on social indicators of deprivation and a wealth of expertise in their use in many local authorities as well as in the academic world (see, for examples of each, Carley 1981, Chapter 7; City of Manchester Planning Department 1982; Greater Manchester Council Planning Department 1985).

The present evaluation therefore must of necessity rely mainly on the extent of the intermediate outputs which we must treat as necessary but not sufficient preconditions for the alleviation of deprivation. We shall none the less have much to say from the experience of our case-studies about the *potential* for the trickle effect to work and about the logic of area designations and the spatial strategy, all of which have far-reaching implications for the extent to which the ultimate goals of the relief of deprivation can be achieved.

EVALUATION

Two central components of the economic regeneration strategy will be evaluated in the pages that follow, using evidence from the four case-studies. The first is the extent to which intermediate aims have been met and what potential they establish for a trickle effect and hence reduction in deprivation. The second is the dependence of the strategy on a number of assumptions about the spatial discreteness of inner cities, the economic activity that goes on in them, and the concentration of deprivation in them.

1   The reach of enterprise

The logic of how the enterprise strategy might impact on deprivation has been detailed in Chapter 4. For the purposes of evaluation of this logic, the relevant intermediate indicators will be the numbers, types and locations of new jobs created, net of any job loss; the extent to which these jobs go to previously unemployed or under-employed local people; and the nature, extent and effectiveness of strategies designed to maximise the take-up of such jobs by local people. (It is worth noting in this respect therefore that the majority of output measures cited by UDCs and such as we have cited in earlier chapters are only very indirectly connected to impact on deprivation.)

There are 35,000 unemployed people within a five-mile radius of the Trafford Centre. Were this scheme to go ahead in anything like the form the original proposal took, it would create 6,500 permanent jobs and a further 2,000 jobs in construction.[1] The permanent jobs would virtually all be in the service sector and the majority as sales personnel. Rather more than one-half would be part-time (see Chapter 8, p. 190). It is not the optimal pattern of job creation on which to base a better future for inner city residents (assuming they got the jobs) but they would be provided at virtually zero cost and they would be a bonus to whatever else was provided in Trafford Park under the auspices of the Development Corporation. Only if the Dumplington site were to be developed for other than retail purposes and to provide more full-time and better-paid jobs would there be opportunity costs involved in the Trafford Centre going ahead. But the development corporation has, of necessity, to take a fairly opportunistic attitude to immigrant investment and since no other large-scale investor has shown much interest in the site, it would seem that the benefits of the Trafford

Centre, imperfect as they are, must be treated as a welcome bonus. The significance of this of course is that there are many potential developments around the country like the Trafford Centre, so located that they could bring some potential employment benefit to deprived areas without public subsidy and without the apparatus of a development corporation or any other form of designation. It is, of course, fortuitous benefit – the 'pure private' example is quite divorced from any inner city policy – but on current showing, it is far from axiomatic that the expensive apparatus of designated agencies performs much better. Indeed, as subsequent discussion shows, neither the London Docklands nor the Trafford Park Development Corporation – nor indeed the Heartlands Agency – have a job creation strategy designed to produce that mix of job types that would create most benefit for their particular local populations. The nearest they come is to offer training for those with the potential to gain from it to compete for such jobs as are produced. But *what* is produced is a matter for chance and the market.

If this sounds like an argument for leaving it all to the private sector and letting inner city policy (and inner city residents) pick up whatever unintended spin-off they can, it isn't. It is to argue however that where there are no good reasons for not allowing such schemes to take place, then neither is there good reason why they should not be permitted and then exploited in such a way as to ensure that the zero- or low-cost jobs they produce go to residents of deprived areas. After all, it would be churlish to expect all inner city benefit to come *only* via designated agencies. And 'pure private' investment *could* be exploited in this way, as we demonstrate in subsequent paragraphs.

The Trafford Centre would (if it were to go ahead) fill just one corner of the designated area of the Trafford Park Development Corporation (although a considerable part of the remaining developable land). Its projected job creation figure of 6,500 therefore makes the target figure of 16,000 for the urban development corporation as a whole look unduly modest. We have already noted however that this figure was adopted almost by default from the original TPIS strategy for Trafford Park and appears to be as notional as most job creation figures cited for development corporations. And the absence of any overall investment or job strategy makes its ethereal nature seem all the more likely. In fact, if the target of 16,000 new jobs were based on a sound assessment of what the development corporation could achieve, it would, after all the efforts and financial investments, leave Trafford Park with 33,000 *fewer* workers than it had at its peak and only 7,000 more than it had at the depths of the depression. Even taking account of changes in technology and manpower requirement, this remains a very modest achievement. It would not be unfair therefore to assume that the

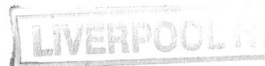

target figure of 16,000 does not represent a realistic assessment of what the development corporation could, or should, achieve over the space of a decade, and that a reasonable expectation would be of a much higher figure. We have to confess however that in the absence of a detailed strategy and with the necessary reliance on opportunism in attracting investment, we are in a no better position to estimate how much in excess of 16,000 a reasonable figure would be. What is possible is to give an approximate idea of the magnitude of the problem: in excess of 45,000 unemployed within a five-mile radius of the Park in 1987 and probably nearer to 50,000 today (mid-1992). As of April 1991, 3,260 new jobs had been created in Trafford Park. No figures are available either for jobs lost or jobs preserved.

If job creation estimates for TPDC seem unduly modest, those for the London Docklands have, as often as not, inhabited the realms of fantasy as Chapter 6 has demonstrated. The 'target' of 200,000 jobs set during the peak of the period of rapid expansion is impossible to relate to the realities of the situation LDDC faced then – let alone the one that confronts it now, in mid-recession (1992). So far as benefit to local people is concerned however, the fantastical nature of the estimates may anyway be of little import because, until relatively recently, the corporation made no pretence that job creation was intended to be for local benefit. 'Regenerating the Docklands' meant just that. It was once more to become an area in which people would want to work and live. *Who* these people were was a matter of indifference. However, this is to encroach on ground that we have covered before. Suffice it to say that the urban development corporations were (and are) promoted by government as the vanguard of inner city policy, and an inner city policy that contains no or few means by which the deprived can be made less deprived is an odd creature. Latterly however, as we have seen, the LDDC has shown itself to be more sensitive to the question of local benefit and the matter of job creation has come under more critical scrutiny. As of August 1991 there was general agreement that the numbers of jobs attracted to Docklands up to the end of 1990 was 41,000 (the figure used by Michael Heseltine in his tenth anniversary speech). The dispute is over the extent to which these jobs represent a net gain of employment in the area and who the beneficiaries of the process have been. Existing firms provided 27,000 jobs in 1981, the year in which LDDC was set up: largely as a result of the development corporation's own relocation policies, these had been reduced to 12,000 by 1990. This loss has been counterbalanced by 17,000 newly created jobs and 24,000 coming in with firms setting up in the Docklands. But the character of these jobs is different – the largest single group is in banking and financial services, jobs which are unlikely to be taken up by local people in any numbers.

There are no job out-turn figures as yet for the Heartlands initiative but there is a specific (more specific than for either development corporation) target for job creation of 20,000 new jobs – a rather more ambitious target, given their relative sizes, than the 16,000 for TPDC. The scale of the potential impact of this target figure, were it to be reached, and if the majority of the jobs went to unemployed local people, can be judged by the fact that in April 1991 there were 5,107 unemployed people in the Aston and Nechells wards of Birmingham (an area approximately corresponding to Heartlands' travel to work zone).

Unless newly created jobs go largely (or at least, in very considerable numbers) to local people who are currently unemployed or under-employed, then the main channel of local benefit from economic re-generation – the 'trickle effect' – is immediately blocked. If, therefore, the government were serious in its aim of reducing deprivation by means of economic regeneration, we should expect policies to maximise this result to be a central part of the entire strategy. In none of the three 'partnership' arrangements that we have examined is this the case, and so far as the Trafford Centre is concerned, the ball would be firmly in the court of Trafford and Salford. There is no reason to believe that the Manchester Ship Canal Company would not have participated in such a strategy (it has a long history of preferring local labour), but up to the time of the planning inquiry – a crucial juncture – no initiative had been forthcoming from the local authorities (Edwards 1987b).

Evidence on local employment benefit is very thin and confined to the two urban development corporations. Trafford Park Development Corporation does not know how many of the 3,260 new jobs in the Park had gone to local people though it was thought that since most of its labour draw area has high unemployment rates, the 'great majority probably had'. Figures produced by consultants for LDDC for local employment benefit from Canary Wharf range, as we have seen, from 1,800 to 21,000. More generally, the proportion of the total work-force of Docklands that lived in the area had declined from 32 per cent in 1981 to 21 per cent in 1986/7 (see p. 110). Given recent developments however, our conclusion must be that if there are any employment gains in Docklands over the first ten years of the devthe development corporation's existence they are marginal and local people have not benefited significantly from them.

Of more significance therefore, given the sparseness of output data so far, is an assessment of what has been and is being done to maximise the extent to which new jobs do go to local people (and which might therefore convey indirect benefit to their dependants). All three of our 'official' agencies had made some efforts at enhancing local job benefit but it cannot be said that any of it was very imaginative or nearly as aggressive as the marketing of enterprise. Other than the (now defunct) possibility of an agreement between LDDC and Olympia & York over the use of local labour at Canary Wharf, almost the entire emphasis so far has been put on training arrangements of one sort or another. And this, as we have seen, came very late in the day at LDDC and has only recently been given any real emphasis in TPDC, where the corporation is supporting or is involved in some ten types of training initiative, has put some forty people through its own tailored schemes and assisted in 580 other places (see p. 93). The London Docklands Development Corporation has already been taken to task for its abysmal record on local benefit both by private consultants and a select committee, and at Trafford Park, steps are only now being taken to head off potentially similar criticisms. On even the most charitable assessment therefore it has to be said that these development corporations have put nowhere near as much energy and enterprise into maximising the benefits for local people of their regeneration activities as they have put into these activities themselves. Indeed, it would not be unfair to say that the *sine qua non* for the relief of deprivation has been relegated to the position of an afterthought.

The position in Heartlands looks potentially brighter, but even there, local benefit is still some way down the agenda and has been mainly the result of spillover from other areas of activity – apart from the housing programme, which we examine in Chapter 10. Employment benefits in the first stage of activity have largely been by-products of the process of physical redevelopment. Perhaps of potentially more interest however is what might have happened at the Trafford Centre. The 'pure private' approach can be exploited for local benefit. Local authorities are not passive spectators of private sector development within or near to their domain and they can, with some will and effort, extract local benefit by 'de-purifying' the process. (It must be added that at the time of the public inquiry, neither Trafford nor Salford had taken steps to exploit the proposed development for local benefit – indeed, as we have seen, Salford opposed it altogether – but that does not mean that it could not be done.)

Strategies for exploiting private development to maximise local benefit through employment fall into three broad categories. Firstly, efforts can be made by local authorities (and, in the case of the Trafford Centre, by the urban development corporation), to make newly created jobs as physically accessible as possible to the main areas of concentration of the unemployed. This may include new road and rail infrastructure (including the Light Rapid Transit) but more importantly, and at far less cost, would be the creation of new bus routes and the bending of existing ones. As two witnesses at the public inquiry into the Trafford Centre pointed out, the addition of 6,500 jobs to the already existing 25,000 in Trafford Park would almost certainly justify such action (Stocks 1987b; Merry 1987). Helping people get to work (and hence helping people to *get* work) ought not to be too taxing an enterprise.

The second component is to maximise the chances of local people getting jobs by making them as competitive as possible in the job market. We have already examined this approach and need not dwell on it here, except to acknowledge that there is considerably more happening on the training front that would be of relevance to the Trafford Centre, than data on the development corporation would lead us to believe. Thus, for example, in the period 1988–9 the Manchester/Salford Partnership put 1,194 people through a variety of training schemes (Manchester/Salford Partnership 1989, Part 3) and in 1987 Salford City Council produced a fairly comprehensive 'plan for jobs' that took on board a wide spectrum of training strategies and which, if implemented with vigour, could have markedly increased the job competitiveness of the local population (Salford City Council 1987b).

The London Docklands DC has eventually woken from its long sleep on the jobs and training issue, graphically described in the evidence given to the House of Commons Employment Committee (see Chapter 6). Training programmes have been considerably expanded and the development corporation now supports 5,000 places. But this figure is still not impressive, especially when set alongside the performance of Merseyside DC, the other 'first generation' UDC, which with only one-fifth of the financial resources supports 7,500 places. An additional area of activity has been compact schemes, described in earlier chapters, in which deals have been made between local schools, employers and the pupils themselves. In Heartlands, compacts involving three local schools have completed their first cycle, with pupils just emerging on to the job market. More ambitious plans in Docklands – the Newham Compact – were linked to the Royal Docks development; the developers, Stanhope Properties, were intending to secure jobs for 5,000 local residents, many of them through developers. This initiative has now been compromised by the withdrawal of the developers as a result of the recession; but it leads us to our next consideration.

The third component is also the most diverse – and potentially the most effective in getting local people into jobs. It consists of a bundle of practices which may loosely be called positive action, designed to 'bend' the competitive employment process in favour of local people. These practices range from the anodyne targeting of job advertisements in localities with concentrations of unemployed people, and the more refined targeting in the ethnic minority press allowed under Section 5(2)d of the Race Relations Act 1976, to the much more effective but illegal use of local labour contracts.

The most effective means of getting local people into the new jobs is the use of quotas enforced through local labour clauses. Such practices however are tainted (not entirely justifiably) by the idea of preferential treatment, and were made illegal under Part I of the Local Government Act 1988 by being classed, along with connections with the nuclear arms industry and trade with South Africa, as 'non commercial considerations'. It was a crass piece of legislative drafting made at a time when the government was indulging its *laissez-faire* tendencies to the full. It denied to the enterprise strategy one of the few (and potentially most effective) instruments it had for increasing regenerative benefits to the locally unemployed. There is, however, some evidence that in this respect, the 1988 Act is something of an embarrassment. Sir Terence Heiser was taken to task over it by the Public Accounts Committee during its hearings on 'Regenerating the Inner Cities' in 1990. When asked whether he was unaware of 'what had happened in the Act', Sir Terence replied:

No, I am fully aware of it. The 1988 Act makes it impossible to put specific conditions in a contract of that kind. We are looking at that with the Department of Employment, because we know of the problems that have been created.

(Heiser 1990: 14)

Subsequently, in describing the Act, Sir Terence noted that 'It was legislation which sought to prohibit what was termed "non commercial" considerations. That is where we got into this particular problem' (Heiser 1990: 19).

It could well be that some form of local labour clause (but not a change in the legislation) will be managed into existence in the relatively near future. It may however relate only to training and not employment *per se*, in which case its 'local benefit' effect would be seriously compromised.

We are deliberating here on what strategies could be used to maximise local employment benefit. The development of the Trafford Centre would not have involved purchase or service contracts between a local authority and the developer and little opportunity in *that* respect to implement local labour clauses. There would however be numerous opportunities during the planning process and the bargaining over permissions for similar sorts of agreement to be written in, quite apart from those provided by local authorities acting as providers of infrastructure.

It seems likely that any agreements entered into at present between developers and local authorities and developers and their tenants in respect of local labour quotas would be unenforceable. That does not mean they need be ineffective. There is much that could be done even within the constraints of the present 1988 Act. Local authorities (and development corporations) could ask for voluntary undertakings on the part of developers to employ as many local people as possible, appealing if necessary to their 'social responsibilities'. There are already many bargains struck during planning negotiations and there is no reason why local benefit should not be one of the counters. (Though it has to be acknowledged that local authorities may be unwilling to trade off against undertakings they know they cannot enforce.) That being said, it remains the case that there is scope and there are opportunities for local government and quasi government agencies to exploit private development for public gain. It is largely a matter of the will, ingenuity and energy to do it. It should be added, however, that (as the Newham case demonstrated) all such initiatives are vulnerable to the effects of economic recession.

The enterprise strategy is too young for any large-scale trickle down effects to be apparent. We do not yet know whether the £1.1bn of public funds so far invested in Docklands and the £68m in Trafford Park have resulted in a lowering of dependency ratios, a reduction in poverty, or indeed a diminution of any of the other components of deprivation. Not only do we not know; the data do not exist from which we might infer an answer. Nor has there been any systematic attempt on the part of any urban development corporation to monitor impact on urban deprivation (though they have no difficulty in producing floorspace figures, investment figures, gearing ratios and the like). In the absence of tailor-made studies (such as time-series surveys in target areas), we shall have to rely on the small area results of the 1991 census to compare with those of 1981. Even then, of course, attributing any measured change in deprivation indicators to the processes of trickle down would be a hazardous enterprise.

What we have been able to do however, in respect of our case studies, is to establish the state (or potential state) of the *preconditions* for any trickle down to occur. And those, as we have seen, are fairly minimal. More damning than the numerical out-turns (in respect of which, for our two urban development corporations, we can only say 'could have done a lot better') is the absence, with the partial exception of Heartlands, of any robust strategy in any of the four examples, for maximising local employment benefit or even of attempting systematically to monitor trickle down effects on urban deprivation. It just has not been taken sufficiently seriously.

Our primary concern has been with the logic of the trickle down effect and the potential for it to happen. The two development corporations we have studied, however, would argue that their contributions to local communities are not confined to such indirect (and possibly capricious) processes but come in the form of direct benefits. The Trafford Park Development Corporation for example would cite its community initiatives programme as a key component of its contribution to community benefit (see pp. 87–8) and LDDC would include the funding of educational schemes, with £13m invested in the Bacons City Technology College and the Tower Hamlets Post-Sixteen College and £1.1m contributed to a computer programme for schools and support for a series of new community facilities – health and community centres and a new town hall for the Isle of Dogs neighbourhood.

Apart from the training component however, these efforts are neither a part of the logic of regeneration nor a necessary component of it. Most are aid in money and kind (and could equally well be done by private or public sectors) and, though they may produce tangible benefit, they do not form a part of the regeneration process with which we are concerned.

2   Area strategies

Inner city policies are spatial policies; they all rely, in some degree or other, on the formal or informal designation of particular areas. The reasons for this are fourfold: it is politically expedient and administratively tidy; the deprived show greater area concentration in urban areas than in rural ones; there is a self-reinforcing effect that compounds the deprivation of the deprived when they are spatially concentrated; and the logic of economic regeneration (which lies at the heart of inner city policy) relies upon the spatial discreteness of economies that can be regenerated. These reasons have already been highlighted in Chapters 3 and 4 in our discussion of enterprise and deprivation; it is time now to return to them in the light of our case-study evidence. There is little more to add about spatial concentration and self-reinforcing effects and they can be despatched fairly quickly. It is around questions of an 'inner city economy' and the discreteness of whatever is to be regenerated that much of the credibility of the enterprise solution revolves.

Most deprived people, as measured by one or more of a range of social indicators, do not live in inner city areas (Holtermann 1975, 1978; Townsend 1976; Robson 1988) and inner city policies will therefore not reach the majority of deprived people. (We did believe this once when deprivation was a residual welfare problem back in the 1960s.) If inner city polices *are* about relieving deprivation therefore (which, given our evaluation so far, is less than self-evident), then their spatial component rests initially on two assumptions: that there are *relative* concentrations of the deprived in inner cities (which is true), and that there is an independent 'neighbourhood effect' that compounds such components of deprivation as exist in an area (which is plausible but not proven – see Chapter 4, p. 69).

In none of the four case-studies was location selected on the grounds of a high relative concentration of the deprived. The Trafford Centre location is where it is because the Manchester Ship Canal Company owned the site and it fulfilled a number of the criteria necessary for a large retail centre. The Trafford Park Urban Development Corporation is where it is because of joint initiatives from the private sector and Trafford Council to rejuvenate the industrial estate. The London Docklands UDC is where it is because Michael Heseltine wanted it, and it is close to the City of London and has lots of water features. Only in the case of Heartlands can it be said that concentrations of deprived people played any part in selecting the 'area of benefit', and even here the choice of site was mainly determined by the development opportunities presented by the existence of a large tract of derelict land (with water features). It is reassuring therefore that all three of the formal schemes (there is no reason why the Trafford Centre should be near concentrations of deprivation) do in fact lie in close proximity to large relative concentrations of the deprived as preceding chapters have shown. Proximity is not the same as accessibility however, and there is no evidence that infrastructure works or 'communal' transport provisions to improve access have in any way been focused to maximise accessibility from deprived areas.[2] Nevertheless, in the minimal sense that each of our case-study 'agencies' has, within its purlieu, large numbers of unemployed people, then they are in the right place. *But* there is a caveat even to this minimal position. The only *entrée* that the enterprise strategy has to that complex of factors that make up deprivation is via employment of the unemployed. Investment therefore needs to be close to concentrations of unemployment. It does not necessarily follow however that concentrations of *other* components of deprivation will coincide with those for unemployment. Indeed, there is evidence that they do not (Holtermann 1975,1978) and to the extent that they do not (or do not always), then we must require of the trickle effect that it operates spatially as well as within and between households and this must necessarily inject an element of ecological dubiety into the logic of the whole process.

The question of an independent self-reinforcing neighbourhood effect remains to be proved. As we noted in Chapter 4, if there is ecological overlap between deprivations it is plausible that the overall effect may be greater than the sum of the parts, but this can only be established at the individual or household level, not at the ecological. However, what we can say that is tangential to this is that none of the 'areas of benefit' for the schemes we have examined constituted neighbourhoods in any substantive sense. We have noted for example that the 'area of benefit' for Heartlands consisted of at least four distinct areas and was not recognisable as an entity by local people. 'Docklands' is a notoriously artificial concept with no clear relationship to the well-defined neighbourhoods in which people live (a 'gigantic cuckoo' is one of the kinder descriptions of the new creation). Similarly, the eight priority areas adopted by the Trafford Park Development Corporation do not coincide with recognisable communities or neighbourhoods. They are in fact defined by ward boundaries. Again Aldridge found in her study of Radford in Nottingham (a key deprivation area for the Nottingham Inner Area Programme) that perceived localities were very small indeed – often just one or two streets – and that 'Radford' was no more than an arbitrary administrative unit (Aldridge and Edwards 1989). It seems likely therefore that if there is any independent neigh- bourhood effect from multiple deprivation, it will not be alleviated to any significant degree by policy effects that impact from and on arbitrarily drawn areas.

THE LOGISTICS OF ENTICEMENT AND THE SPATIAL SHIBBOLETH

Inner city policy *needs* discrete spatial areas with defined boundaries; it cannot, in its present form, operate in any other way. There have to be designated areas within which the enticements to the private sector are operative and outwith which they are not. (The same goes for the urban programme of course; the 75 per cent central government grant applies only within defined areas, though they may be drawn more widely and flexibly than urban development areas.) We have already noted how the contingencies of such policies can elevate the spatial aspect of inner cities to an *idée fixe*. There are sound political and administrative reasons why this should be so. Area designations were in part a reaction to the failure of the 'scattergun' approach of the original urban programme (see Edwards and Batley 1978); it is potentially easier to demonstrate results when efforts are concentrated on a defined area, and the mechanics of the leverage approach demand designation. It is less evident that the reduction of urban deprivation is best served however by such an emphasis on the spatial. We shall use the remainder of this chapter to evaluate the spatial emphasis of the enterprise strategy and will do so in respect of three issues that have emerged from the case-studies. The first is the idea of an inner city economy. The second is the contingent notion that there is something *to be* regenerated in a process of reversing history. The third concerns the question of whether investment must be *in* the inner city to be of benefit to it.

'Regenerating inner city economies' has been the leitmotiv of inner city policy for more than a decade. The enterprise strategy depends on it, and once the root cause of the inner city problem had been diagnosed (as long ago as 1975 or thereabouts) as the collapse of these economies, logic (but not necessarily sense) dictated their rejuvenation as the solution. Yet they remain chimerical. There is economic activity (some) in inner city areas but that is not the same as an inner city economy which, as we have noted in an earlier chapter, though undefined, must mean (if it means anything) relatively self-contained local economies which happen to be in inner city areas. And this presumably implies economic activity from which the majority of local residents gain their livelihood and back into which they recycle their income, thus supporting a service sector which in part at least will support productive activity. If such relatively discrete economies once existed there is little evidence that they do now, even in a debilitated form that could be regenerated. It is difficult therefore to see what it is that is to be regenerated unless, when boiled down to its essentials, it is not an inner city economy but economic activity in inner city areas. If it is – and this seems to be the most likely interpretation – then an altogether different question arises. Inner city economies, given their relatively self-contained nature as characterised above, must necessarily be in the inner city. If, on the other hand, we are talking about economic activity that is available to inner city residents, there is no necessary reason why it has to be located *in* the inner city – and several good reasons why it should not.

It is far from convincing therefore that there ever was a discrete inner city economy in any of our three locations whilst it can be said that there used to be more employment there than there is now (which has potentially quite different policy implications). The London Docklands Development Corporation for example is not regenerating an old economy; it is creating a new and quite different one – one from which local residents are less likely to benefit. There may, in the nineteenth century, have been something that looked rather like an inner city economy in Heartlands, but it is too close to the city centre to sustain a semi-independent economy now and the investment that will be attracted there will have more national, international or city-wide links than it will with the arbitrarily bounded area of that name. Only in Trafford Park is there a 'natural' area to be regenerated. But this never was an 'inner city economy' (in the sense that we have defined it) because it never had more than a nominal population (600 at most). There is no pretence therefore of regenerating an inner city economy in Trafford Park. The aim must be the more straightforward one of reinstating the Park, at least in part to the role it played for more than half a century as Greater Manchester's economic larder. The danger will be (for inner city residents at least) that the larder will be stocked with goods that are of little use to them.

But somewhere along the line the idea of a spatially discrete inner city economy which provided the life-blood for the inner city area became enshrined as canon. Boundaries could be drawn around it; it could be regenerated as though it existed in both spatial and economic isolation; investment levered into it would have a regenerating effect (and the people living in it would be 'entrepreneurialised'). But not investment on the other side of the boundary. And so there developed an entire logic of enterprise-led regeneration with new, single-minded bodies to effect it, boundaries within which they could exercise their new powers and a logistics of enticement to make it all work.

All of this might not matter (it might not work either – in fact it won't if the purpose is to recreate the irredeemable) were it not for the potentially damaging effects on areas outside the boundaries of benefit. Just as the enterprise zones created zones of depression outside their walls, so might urban development corporations and urban development agencies such as Heartlands suck in investment to the detriment of surrounding areas.[3] And the irony of this is that the surrounding areas are just as likely to be areas of deprivation as that within the arbitrarily drawn boundary. A clear example of the fatuity of this dogma of spatial enticement was the nature of much of the opposition at the public inquiry into the Trafford Centre development that we described in some detail in Chapter 8. Whatever the merits and flaws of the development (and there were both), to oppose it on the grounds that it would either damage the city centres of Salford, Trafford and Manchester or the inner city areas of Greater Manchester (or both) was to fly in the face of logic – and of government policy. If a major job-creating development in an urban development corporation was going to damage the inner cities, one is left wondering what the UDC is doing there in the first place (and what all this business of urban regeneration is all about).

The opposition however was based not on the 'economic larder' theory but on a reification of the 'inner city economy'. In short, to be of benefit to the inner city, investment had to be *in* it ('it' again being defined arbitrarily). There appear to be no grounds to support this assertion, other than an obeisance to the reversing history hypothesis. Gone are the days when local firms could support the local population and be supported by them – changes in manufacturing and technology have seen to that. There is no longer a case for the close intermingling of production and residential functions (if there ever was, other than to minimise the time the worker was not at his bench). And there is no evidence that, given as much un-constrained choice, the inner city resident would still want, or enjoy being part of, that 'hustle and bustle on a human scale' than would her suburban counterpart (or Mr Heseltine for that matter). It is, after all, a peculiarly anthropological view.

Would it not make more sense therefore (and probably be more in accord with the wishes of inner city residents) to redevelop deprived and run-down areas as environmentally pleasant and safe residential areas with good quality housing and services, such as would be attractive to anthropologists and Mr Heseltine, and concentrate job-creating investment in segregated but accessible locations? Trafford Park could provide a model for this; it does not pretend to be anything other than an industrial estate, and no one need live there. Neither the London Docklands, nor Heartlands, to the extent that they are trying to recreate inner city economies, fit this mould. They are in pursuit of something altogether more ambitious, and in that particular aim they will fail. It might have turned out to be more productive of benefit to the deprived had they kept it simple.

NOTES

1   These are definitive figures should the scheme go ahead. They are far less speculative therefore than estimates in urban development corporations.
2   This is not to say that steps to improve accessibility have not generally been taken, especially in the two development corporations, or that people in the deprived areas will not benefit thereby.
3   In Trafford Park, as we have seen, the enterprise zones *within* the urban development corporation have had the same effect.

10 Social policies for the inner city

VARIATIONS ON EMPOWERMENT

At various stages in our description of the different initiatives that have been undertaken since the new phase of urban policy began in 1977, we have paused to ask the question: who has benefited? The previous chapter sets out some ways in which the economic consequences of these new enterprise-led developments have impacted on the areas in which they have been conducted, their inhabitants and in some cases neighbouring localities.

In this chapter, we explore ways in which social policies have emerged that relate to the other indices of deprivation that we identified in Chapter 3: environmental conditions, the delivery of services and availability of opportunities for individual and collective self-advancement. In doing so we will necessarily have to address the issue of dependency and the notion – so influential in the policies of the 1980s – that the key to regeneration lies in a change of values among inner city residents.

In doing so, we will also briefly review the range of attempts that have been made to construct alternative bases for inner city social policies around the themes of partnership through the participation of local people and what is often inelegantly called the 'bottom-up' approach to regeneration through locality-based initiatives intended to empower the residents themselves.

The recurrent reproach, through this and previous phases of policy, has been that whatever approach has been adopted by the policy makers it is the people of the localities selected for the new interventions who have gained least from them. Do the new policies – especially those introduced by the Conservative government after 1981 under the banner of 'enterprise' – escape this reproach? In particular, has the concept of local people as individual consumers profiting from resources that trickle down to them as a result of economic regeneration to construct their own solutions – 'empowerment' in an altogether different sense – proved to be more effective as a way of improving the circumstances of people who live in cities?

The primary emphasis on economic regeneration first introduced in Peter Shore's White Paper of 1977 carried with it as an appendage a commitment to involve local communities in the partnership now proposed. 'Involving local people', the authors proclaimed, 'is both a necessary means to the regeneration of the inner areas and an end in its own right' (Department of the Environment 1977e, para 34). However, the rationale for this partnership and the form that it should take was heavily influenced by the turbulent history of other programmes that had once had more far-reaching ambitions in this direction. The story of the most controversial of these, the community development projects (CDPs), has frequently been told (we have summarised it in Chapter 2 but see also Marris 1982; Higgins *et al.* 1983; Loney 1983). For present purposes, it is sufficient to say that the breakdown of confidence and communications between the CDP teams and the government department that sponsored them (the Home Office, which took the lead on inner city policy up to 1976), leading eventually to mutual repudiation, left lasting scars on both sides. This in turn ensured that community-based approaches would in future be viewed with extreme caution in Whitehall; and that functionally no initiative would again be allowed the degree of autonomy enjoyed by the CDP projects.

In fact, although CDPs carried 'community' in their title, the emphasis in their later work had moved a long way from the focus on intensive work within the small highly-deprived areas that the teams had initially been established to regenerate. Instead, the major theme of their later work (as we saw in Chapter 2) had been on the structural changes in the regional and national economy that had led to the decline of the areas on which the teams were ostensibly working; and among the major causes of this decline the teams identified the failure of local authorities and their members and professional staff to measure up to the nature and extent of the underlying problems (see Community Development Project 1977a, b).

In advancing their critique, the CDP teams were able to draw on a large stockpile of ammunition accumulated in the great planning battles of the late 1960s and early 1970s. The rationalist model of strategic planning that had then been recently introduced had carried within it consultation as an ingredient (see Skeffington Report 1969). But this had rapidly come to be derided as 'incorporation' and swept aside by demands for the exercise of full-scale control over the planning process by the community. These developments were seen at their most dramatic in the struggle over the redevelopment of the Covent Garden market (Anson 1981) and in their most long-lasting form in the London Docklands, where the efforts of community-based groups to become involved in the process of replanning precipitated by the closure of the docks began in earnest in the response to the Travers Morgan plan (1973) and achieved some measure of success during the later 1970s before they were abruptly cut short by the declaration of the London Docklands Development Corporation (Marris 1982, and see Chapter 6 of this volume).

All these different responses originally had in common a hostility to the local authority-centred approach which had up to then been the dominant form in inner city initiatives (Higgins *et al.* 1983) and drew on all the accumulated distrust of local government's past record in planning and housing. This distrust was, if anything, intensified by the change of style introduced in the new local government system established under the Walker Act (1972), particularly in the strategic authorities – the new metropolitan counties and the GLC – including corporate planning and planned programme budgeting systems. In a polemical analysis of these trends, John Benington of Coventry CDP denounced them as the epitome of the process by which 'Local Government Becomes Big Business' (Community Development Project 1975). And in one of their concluding reports, the joint teams, having (in Peter Marris's phrase) dismissed 'a decade of inner city anti-poverty programmes with contempt for their repetitive futility' (Marris 1982: 32), proposed instead that

> the 'regional problem' and the 'inner city problem' were themselves the products of a certain mode of capitalist development and that it was inadequate to deal with them by merely rejigging varieties of incentive or by positive discriminatory practices . . . simply planning the infrastructure whilst leaving the underlying industrial and economic structures to the whim of the private entrepreneur had been proved to be no solution.
>
> (Community Development Project 1977b: 95)

Against this background, it is perhaps not surprising that the 1977 White Paper should have been so cautious in the treatment that it gave to the scope for community involvement-choosing rather than to stress the potential contribution of voluntary organisations whose role in social policy was in the course of being rehabilitated (Wolfenden Report 1978). Although its authors accepted the diagnosis of economic decline as the major cause of the inner cities problems, the remedies advanced were seen in terms of a partnership in which the local authorities would continue to be key actors. As the White Paper puts it,

> Local authorities are the natural agencies to tackle inner area problems. They are democratically accountable bodies; they have long experience of running local services, most of which no other body could provide as effectively or as sensitively to local needs.
>
> (Department of the Environment 1977e, para 31)

So, to the extent that it remained a policy objective, local community involvement was an appendage to the activities of local government – who were expected to carry their local populations (and occasional electorates) with them in the implementation of the new initiatives being designed by the partnership between the different tiers of government.

As we have already seen, the incoming Conservatives saw matters differently. Although the structures established by Shore were left in place and the basic diagnosis – which went back not to CDP but to the inner area studies produced by consultants commissioned by his Conservative predecessor Peter Walker – was accepted, the emphasis in implementation was entirely different. Like the CDP teams, but for quite different reasons, the Conservative government saw local government not as providing solutions but as a major part of the problem. But if involving local authorities was no longer a policy objective, it followed that should involvement of community continue to be a policy goal (even a subordinate one), then other ways of reaching local populations would have to be devised.

NEW SOCIAL POLICIES

The enterprise alternative

The goals of the new approach to inner city policy were first codified in the 1980 legislation which provided the basis for establishing the urban development corporations. As we saw in Chapter 2, the role of the UDCs was quite narrowly demarcated, but did include in Section 136 (2) the duty to ensure that 'housing and social facilities are available to encourage people to live and work in the area' – what was referred to by the civil servant responsible before the House of Commons Employment committee as 'a very small point at the very end' (see Chapter 6).

The priority given in the gloss has already been noted; perhaps more so, the fact that the legislation encourages people *to* live, not *who* live in the areas chosen. This reflected Michael Heseltine's own emphasis as Minister then responsible that

> the right use of the extra funding would be not only to help the existing community but also to entice back, by improving the fabric and commercial environment, the more enterprising who had left town and taken their skills and energy with them.
>
> (Heseltine 1987: 138)

Heseltine and his colleagues were quite emphatic in their belief that local authorities in deprived inner city areas had not succeeded in catering for the aspirations either of their existing population or those who had departed and might return. As the pattern of Conservative social policy began to develop over the course of the 1980s, two complementary themes emerged: firstly, the progressive reduction in the executive role of local authorities; and secondly, the emphasis on 'empowerment' of individuals and their families, both through extension of the role of the market and by encouragement of individual self-help. Both themes are reflected in the development of inner city policy and the instruments devised to implement it.

The general downgrading of the role of local government hardly needs further underlining here, since it is one of the most conspicuous features of Conservative policy (see Chapters 2 and 3). In this context, it is perhaps most significant in abolishing or substantially curtailing the access that inhabitants of inner city areas have had to policy making and implementation through their right to participate in the democratic electoral process. The fact that the vast majority of them have not in the past chosen to exercise that right does not in principle detract from the force of the point. These developments mean that, to take the most obvious example, inhabitants of those parts of the three London boroughs that fall within the operational area of the London Docklands Development Corporation who are aggrieved by planning decisions cannot pursue their grievances through their local elected member; the line of accountability is broken.

The government answers these criticisms in two ways: firstly, by asserting that local authorities (especially those in inner city areas which have almost all been under Labour control during the 1980s) have ceased to provide an authentic reflection of the wishes of local people and have thereby forfeited their right to be considered representative. Secondly, that there are valid alternative ways of reflecting local wishes and allowing local people a share in decision taking. So the objective has been, as Heseltine defined it, to 'push power out beyond local government and into the hands of the people whom it is elected to serve' (Heseltine 1987: 132).

These conclusions are reflected in some – though not all – of the general policies adopted over the course of the 1980s (for example, sale of housing to tenants, local management of schools and encouragement of private pensions schemes) and were applied through specific inner city policies. The question has been how best to present them in the context of a general emphasis on economic regeneration as the principal objective of policy and on the private sector as the means through which it will be achieved. Moreover, here (and even more so in the USA) this policy emphasis ('privatism') has been reinforced by a deliberate attempt to switch government spending wherever possible out of social programmes and into those that directly support economic regeneration. This was vividly reflected in the performance of the senior DoE witness before the House of Commons Employment Committee, with his continual stress on the role of UDCs as bringing 'a single-minded approach to physical regeneration' (House of Commons Employment Committee 1988b: Q92) and the same official's subsequent rebuke to London Docklands Development Corporation when it attempted to take a new and broader approach (see Chapter 6 – although it should be added that there has been some modification of attitudes since then).

Delivering new policies

There are three detectable strands in the attempt to develop new social policies as they have emerged during the course of the 1980s which can be credibly presented as bringing direct benefit to local people. We can label them 'trickle down', 'developer's social conscience' and 'public sector substitution'.

The issue of the effectiveness of 'trickle down' as a means of enhancing the economic circumstances of local residents formed a major theme of discussion in Chapter 9. The point to emphasise here is that benefits for those living locally are presented as part of the general gains made by the re-establishment of an 'enterprise culture' and the national economic revival achieved as a result. Apart from the purely economic element it is proposed that there is a recovery of a sense of common purpose and collective morale through casting off dependency – which in turn is per-ceived as one of the major obstacles to inner city regeneration.

The essence of this approach is captured, for what it is worth, in the sequence of 'glossies' issued after the repackaging of urban policy in response to the then Prime Minister's 1987 pledge. The change in attitudes (she opines in her introduction to the first of these) will provide inner city residents with 'more opportunities to share in the new prosperity' through 'rediscovering the sense of civic pride that once united residents and business' (Cabinet Office 1988). In the following year, 'rapidly falling unemployment' was cited as evidence that local people were indeed bene-fiting; and greater involvement of local residents than in the past was promised, together with 'participation of community groups in plans for the development of their areas' (Department of the Environment 1989b). In the third year of the programme, *People in Cities* (1990) stressed 'the new hope and confidence which enterprise in the cities is giving people – and the contribution they can make to ensuring that the spirit of enterprise continues to rise', although 'there remain areas, often quite small, where the local people have not yet been able to take advantage fully – where their self-confidence remains low and their expectations and aspirations modest' (Department of the Environment 1990b).

In the fourth year of the programme (1991), economic recession had taken hold, Britain was bottom of the European growth league and unemployment was rising sharply. There was a new Prime Minister. No report was issued.

In default of any substantial evidence of continued benefits for inner urban areas flowing from the effects of national economic policies, the likelihood of attitudes towards the enterprise culture being systematically transformed in a positive direction now seems somewhat remote. Indeed, the opposite may be the case: the return of mass unemployment must put at risk much of the locally-based work on economic regeneration, particularly the attempt to revive local economies through support for small businesses and work with ethnic minorities, who are always more vulnerable to unemployment in recessions. The effect on motivation is bound to be substantial, although particular local circumstances may still produce different outcomes.

However, there is a second source of possible social benefits for inner city residents in the spin-offs from the operation of industrialists and developers, either individual enterprises operating within particular areas or collectively, as part of the general process of developing a climate of corporate social responsibility. The history of the evolution of corporate responsibility in the United States and its applications to the problems of inner cities there is traced in Barnekov *et al.* (1989). Having burned their fingers on involvement in federal social programmes during the war on poverty in the 1960s, the powerful coalitions of commercial interests that had developed switched their attention in the 1970s with the encouragement of federal government to explicitly economic objectives – characteristically, setting up local urban development trusts as vehicles for partnership, attracting city and federal funds. In the process, industry became accustomed to the notion that a (rather thin) slice of the action would be expected of them in the form of community benefit.

In the course of the scramble to exchange ideas across the Atlantic at the beginning of the 1980s (see Chapter 4) some of these notions were stirred into the pudding that Heseltine's joint public–private sector group (FIG) was cooking up together as part of the exercise in redirecting policy towards a stronger private sector lead. Business in the Community (BiC) energetically pursued the same theme, with royal patronage as an extra come-on, when the Prince of Wales gave his personal blessing to the notion of corporate responsibility. Social programmes proliferated: secondments, grants, setting up of community trusts. Pilkingtons in St Helens were the pioneers here; their acceptance of a share of responsibility for social outcomes in the town in which they were the dominant employers 'greatly impressed' Michael Heseltine when he first saw it after the 1979 election and he subsequently championed the trust model energetically as a basis for action (Heseltine 1987: 165).

As a result of this ministerial promotion, this process eventually began to take the form of explicit involvement in new inner city initiatives. One of the most interesting episodes of this kind was the creation of the Stockbridge Village Trust, an event vividly captured in the account given by Gerry Stoker (see Brindley *et al.* 1989).

The origins of the Stockbridge episode lay in Michael Heseltine's presence on Merseyside, during the period of his personal involvement with the task force set up after the 1981 disturbances. Asking to see the worst local authority housing estate in the area, he was taken to Cantril Farm in Knowsley, an overspill housing estate designed and built by Liverpool City Council for former inhabitants of slum clearance areas in Everton. Following his visit in June 1982, he asked his former housing advisor, Tom Baron, to draw up a scheme for private-sector regeneration of the estate. Baron's plan was to create a non-profit-making trust to which the estate could be transferred by the authority. The Abbey National Building Society and Barclays Bank were persuaded to invest; and the developer Laurie Barratt (shortly to be Sir Laurie) to act as sole contractor for the demolition, rehabilitation and new construction envisaged. Cantril Farm was duly reborn as Stockbridge Village Trust, with a management structure incorporating representatives of the major stakeholders (a 50:50 public–private sector division) and one representative from the community. A strong management style was adopted with an emphasis on action rather than accountability; local people were invited to 'share the vision' rather than to participate in realising it.

Within two years of its creation, the trust was on the brink of financial catastrophe precipitated by slack financial management and the withdrawal of Barratts from the 'flagship' scheme – rehabilitation of the central tower blocks. As Stoker analysed it: 'the trust's problem was that while the public sector contribution was forthcoming the funds from the private sector were not' (Brindley *et al.* 1989: 148). Costs had been seriously underestimated; and Barratts had taken a decision, based on commercial considerations, to pull out. Their attitude was the precise opposite of that taken by Barclays and Abbey National, who had invested not in a commercial undertaking but a high-profile political initiative with direct ministerial involvement and strong emphasis on community benefits.

Stockbridge was eventually rescued by a substantial investment of additional public funds to which (since it was allocated through the urban programme) the local authority had to make a sizeable contribution. This outcome wholly negated Heseltine's initial operating assumption – 'it would be interesting to see', he had observed, 'what can be done here without recourse to public funds' (Heseltine 1987: 156) – which may explain the blandly misleading account he gives in his own book. More important, it suggests that there are limits to what can be realistically expected from the 'give a damn' approach through motivated businessmen. To put it in their own terms, when the financial going gets tough, the tough get going – out of the project. Most important of all, it suggests that reliance on the private sector alone to deliver supplementary social benefit may be misconceived (a point to which we return in the next section).

Certainly, the behaviour of transatlantic firms drawn into investment in the British inner city programme by the incentives offered, who have much longer experience of this kind of operating environment, suggests that while they are quite willing to strike the necessary bargains, they will not allow this process to obscure the main purpose of investment: company profits. The developers involved in the largest Docklands scheme – Olympia & York (Canary Wharf) – gave evidence to the House of Commons Employment Committee on their practices. While they were clearly on their best behaviour, witnesses were clear about what Olympia & York called in their written evidence 'the value of establishing good relations with the local populations' and making 'their contribution to a complex and fragile social and built environment', with the aim of 'reviving the economy of an area of London with a vibrant community life' (House of Commons Employment Committee 1988b: 242, 246). In a practical sense (see Chapter 6), this boiled down to a commitment to recruit local labour where appropriate skills existed or training could be provided; the developers' representatives politely evaded the attempt of the Select Committee's chairman to persuade them to offer a more far-reaching and imaginative definition of 'community gain', although they have sub-sequently embarked on a number of new initiatives, including an arts programme aimed at 'creating a strong cultural life in a largely corporate setting' (*Docklands News*, August 1991). Their example has been imitated by other major Docklands private sector stakeholders, like News International, who have also established trusts whose brief includes support for community schemes.

Nevertheless, the balance of experience suggests that any systematic enhancement of community benefit from development-led regeneration policies would have to come from the third direction identified earlier: 'public sector substitution'. Consultants – always a sensitive weather-vane – had begun to indicate from the mid-1980s in the reports commissioned by LDDC that there were deficiencies in their programmes (notably in training and job creation) that would have to be made good – especially given the continued hostility of groups in the community. Clearly, if the operation was to continue to be management-led and the style non-participative, consumer satisfaction would be correspondingly more important.

Some of the Mark Two UDCs set up shortly afterwards also began by distancing themselves from the commercial opportunity-led approach of LDDC – perhaps in part because the option to imitate their approach did not exist; one of the distinguishing marks of those that took a different approach (Trafford Park DC was not initially one of them) was to be their involvement in a wider range of executive programmes, though not necessarily in an executive capacity. As the deputy chair of the Black Country DC, Jean Denton, summed it up in a torrent of words for the Select Committee:

> We have knowledge which is not available. We also have focus. We are not tasked on the health situation, we are not highways, we are not education other than where we can help and where we can see – let me not pretend we do not see education as key to almost anything you go near long term. We are tasked to regenerate. It means that the resources they have can be better used and we are also not tasked to be reelected, we have only one measure of success.
>
> (House of Commons Employment Committee 1988b: 266)

For the powers of UDCs, as the DoE was never tired of reminding them, were very limited – and physical regeneration was a heavy call on the funds provided up front by government within the urban block. Corporations consequently edged cautiously and with limited commitment into funding social programmes.

But the same was not true of some of the other new agencies created in the course of the 1980s, in particular the inner city task forces. As we saw in Chapter 2, task forces have been managed from the Department of Trade and Industry and are principally concerned with employment generation and support for small firms. But apart from jobs and training (including work with schools) their briefs have also come to include environmental improvement and crime prevention – both areas where they come into direct competition with local authorities. In addition, their function of stimulating new activity, raising awareness and (most important of all) drawing in funds from other government agencies has given them access to a wider array of resources and the opportunity to experiment. Operating with a direct line through a small central unit to ministers, task forces are also able to reduce time taken to approve and fund projects: compare the detailed scrutiny and lengthy delays that have characterised the Department of the Environment's management of the Urban Programme (Audit Commission 1989).

Task forces therefore find themselves operating on local authorities' patches, sometimes with overlapping briefs and dealing direct with a wide range of community organisations. Several of them have made a particular point of developing links with ethnic minority organisations. The initial consultants' report on Handsworth commented that if one feature of their work had to be singled out, it would be the task force's ability 'to target the benefits of the policy to specific disadvantaged groups – to a degree which is unparalleled in other government policy areas concerned with economic development' (PA/Cambridge Economic Consultants 1991a). To this extent, the government was establishing a link that bypassed local authorities and dealt direct with groups in need in ways that development-led policies (as the task force evaluation delicately implies) did not. It seems clear that at the outset the 'barely hidden agenda' (as Robin Thompson puts it) was to 'show that local government is a largely redundant element in the regeneration process' (*Samizdat*, July/August 1990), although the practical lessons of the experience of four years of operation in the field is the opposite: 'that Task Forces have a greater impact and are most cost-effective when they have the active positive support of their respective local authorities' (PA/Cambridge Economic Consultants 1991a: vi).

But the task force's work was almost wholly undertaken from public funds – the amount of private funding 'leveraged' has been 'low by the standards of some other urban policy instruments' (PA/Cambridge Economic Consultants 1991a, 1991b: para 3.3.8). With the spectacular (and short-lived) exception of the Merseyside task force, which came from a different stable (the DoE) and operated under direct patronage of the Secretary of State (for which see Parkinson and Duffy 1984), the task force style could also be seen as an adaptation and extension of the public sector entrepreneurialism that had come to characterise the more successful elements in the activities of the inner city partnerships and programme authorities.

Much of the work on social programmes led by the public sector has simply been a continuation of what has been undertaken through partnership inner area programmes and in the Urban Programmes since 1977. Despite the criticisms Michael Heseltine made of them on taking office, no major structural changes have been made in this system. However, there have been substantial shifts in the content of programmes, from social to economic and revenue expenditure to capital (for the detail of which see Chapter 2) and also in the ethos. In particular, the DoE has been concerned to favour those projects that embody the values of entrepreneurship and wherever possible are not managed within the public sector. The voluntary sector have been to some extent the beneficiaries of this change of emphasis; the ministerial guidelines issued after a review of procedures in 1985 stress that social projects supported through the programme should 'encourage the development of more cost-effective and more economic ways of alleviating the effects of urban deprivation and tacking new social problems' (Department of the Environment 1985, para 15) and add that voluntary 'or other' groups may be particularly well placed to develop projects that 'embody a new approach to problems or fill gaps in existing services'.

But voluntary sector and community groups have had at the same time to contend with some more far-reaching difficulties brought about by the progressively greater stringency of the financial regime imposed on local government through the 1980s. These problems have come to a head in many partnership and programme authority areas when the time has come to transfer time-expired projects from the Urban Programme to main service programme funding. This is one among many illustrations that one of the implications for inner urban areas of changed policy priorities under the Conservatives has been a substantial reduction in the sums available to sustain major social programme activities. This process is seen most clearly in the cuts made in housing investment programmes and social services and education budgets of local authorities during the 1980s, which led one local authority association to comment sourly that 'if this process is not reversed and if a true urban policy is not developed, local government will not be there to respond if things go wrong in future' (Association of Metropolitan Authorities 1988).

Against this background, it is perhaps surprising that alternative inner city policies with direct impact on inhabitants of inner areas should have been sustainable. But they have been and could be divided into two categories. Firstly, there have been the activities of the original partnership and programme authorities, together with those other fifty-seven local authorities in whose areas the Urban Programme functions. These are still employing public funds to implement local authority-led programmes whose content is intended to be related to local needs. In addition, there are activities funded under Section 11 of the 1966 Local Government Act, in its new form. This still relates specifically to ethnic minorities but has now been modified to bring it alongside the new programmes launched in the course of the 1980s. Taken together, these programmes offer the basis of an alternative approach not entirely superseded by subsequent experience, based on the original 1977 concept of public sector partnership with some links to local community groups. The attitude of the government towards this type of approach has been ambiguous: first critical, then indifferent, and latterly a sudden attempt to import the values of the enterprise culture by compelling local authorities to compete publicly for their share of funds within a fixed budget, in the so-called Inner City Challenge.

The second category consists of new programmes launched during the course of the last decade from outside government and specifically directed at benefiting the inhabitants of inner city areas. These in turn fall into two sub-categories: those that represent an adaptation of the government's approach and which although not explicitly designed as part of the range of enterprise policies are none the less broadly consistent with them. Heartlands (see Chapter 7) is one key example of this type of initiative, which has clear implications for the resident community; another, more fully developed, is the GEAR project that was promoted by the Scottish Office through the Scottish Development Agency (SDA) in the East End of Glasgow, after 1976. This is now formally wound up and has been the subject of an outside review (Donnison and Middleton 1987).

In the second category are schemes that have been launched by local authorities in direct opposition to the government's policies. Much of the impetus behind these developments comes from the inheritors of the critical tradition descending from CDP and described at the beginning of this chapter. The paradox is that from having been among local government's severest critics they have become its most fervent defenders – a process not unconnected with the fact that many of those concerned found work there when a series of inner city authorities fell under control of what can be loosely categorised as the New Urban Left. Much of the work done by these authorities was on local economic development and falls outside the scope of this chapter. But some of the schemes promoted by left-wing Labour authorities were specifically directed at empowerment – in precisely the opposite sense to that employed by the government – particularly those developed by the GLC after 1981 under the heading of 'popular planning'. While much of this work was undertaken as part of an attempt to block the implementation of initiatives being undertaken by the Conservatives, specifically in Docklands, where the GLC helped to fund many of the community-based groups who formed the principal opposition to the LDDC (see Chapter 6), the concept was also employed in a positive way. In at least one case, the redevelopment of the Coin Street site on the south bank of the Thames by Waterloo Station, it was worked through to completion. The original intention had been to use the site for a large hotel; but the recession of the early 1970s led to the abandonment of the original scheme and eventually to the first of a lengthy series of public inquiries. As a result, Michael Heseltine, by then Secretary of State for the Environment, refused to give permission either for 'massive and over-dominant' office proposals or for housing plans, put forward by community groups, that 'failed to exploit the employment potential of the site'. A further round of planning and negotiation ended in stalemate, broken when the potential developers sold their interest to the GLC, itself by then on the verge of extinction, who then turned the land over to the Society for Cooperative Dwellings and a newly-formed non-profit company, Coin Street Community Builders, who have since been engaged in implementing the plans drawn up by local community groups. The housing element will be owned and managed by tenants in seven separate housing cooperatives (Brindley *et al.* 1989; Ward 1989).

Coin Street is an example of redevelopment of a substantial – and valuable – site in a city centre location being conducted according to different principles. Most important, it is a clear case of an initiative that originated within a local community and owes its form to the priorities that emerged as a result of local people's lengthy struggle to obtain control over the processes of development. The outcomes in terms of social programmes and the extent and types of benefit achieved for the local community are clearly relevant to any discussion of the extent of community gain achieved by different approaches (Brindley *et al.* 1989). Self-help as an alternative option does now have some demonstrable achievements to report (Ward 1989).

Appraisal

Some general principles

From the discussion in the first half of this chapter it should now be evident that the activities which have been taking place over the course of the 1980s in the inner cities, which either involve or impact directly on the welfare of localities and their inhabitants and the problems experienced under the general heading of deprivation, as we defined them in Chapter 3, can be sorted into three broad groups. These are: first, the policies promoted by the Conservative government which are (at least in theory) private sector led – the 'enterprise initiatives'; second, the survivors of previous public sector-based programmes, together with a few new central government schemes – 'public partnerships'; and third, a small group of new schemes either promoted by local authorities or evolved within communities as self-help initiatives over the course of the decade: 'popular planning'.

In practice, the boundaries between these different categories is permeable; the enterprise approach rests heavily on public sector funding and logistic support; public sector partnership is increasingly informed by the values of the market as local authorities compete for private investment (and now public funds) and adjust their style to improve their attractions – what is sometimes called 'municipal mercantilism'; and popular planning often proves to have contained a strong dose of old-fashioned top-down direction alongside its aspirations to plan 'bottom-up'. Nevertheless, the core of each group is sufficiently distinctive to justify an attempt at comparisons between them in terms of the different methods that they have adopted to promote social programmes that will meet local needs and address problems of deprivation.

There are, however, some further issues about the terms in which any appraisal can be conducted. Most of the new initiatives introduced by the Conservatives – in particular the UDCs – have stated objectives which are often (as we have seen in earlier chapters) set out in quantified terms. However, as we pointed out in Chapter 9, very few of these objectives impinge directly upon the issues now being explored; they mostly relate to success in attracting private sector investment and the immediate commercial consequences of such investment. Where there are goals that can be convincingly linked to the welfare of the present inhabitants of designated inner city areas they tend to be secondary, and the extent to which benefit is conferred on the existing inhabitants is problematic. Nor do they tend to figure in formal evaluations of performance. The key examples here would be creation of jobs and construction of new housing. Furthermore, in the UDCs – especially the two we have examined, Trafford Park and London Docklands – the new schemes that are introduced have been development (or rather developer) led and there is no master plan; it is therefore difficult to measure success even against these criteria.

Latterly, changes of direction have meant that programmes with a specific social content are being promoted (by some UDCs) which will be susceptible to appraisal, in due course. In addition, some of the other enterprise initiatives are public sector led as well as resourced and are more susceptible to appraisal in terms of their stated objectives. A number of such appraisals conducted by consultants either for the lead government departments concerned or the development corporations exist, and within limits provide a basis for judgements on their effectiveness in terms of their stated goals. However, because of the limited way in which objectives are still defined, the evidence from these studies is in most cases marginal to any attempt to sum up the gains and losses to the welfare of local inhabitants.

So in general, the claims made on behalf of all this group of 'enterprise' initiatives that they have made a significant impact in this area rest on the general propositions advanced (e.g. in the glossies) to have 'created a climate of enterprise' and 'improved the image of the area'. These achievements are in turn held to lead to improved opportunities for the individual inhabitants of such areas in terms of job opportunities and lifestyle, should they be motivated to take advantage of them. It is recognised that in some cases past lack of motivation may be due to 'a degree of market failure' (to use the words of the evaluators of the Task Forces, PA/Cambridge Economic Consultants), which is reflected in circumstances in the area itself. National economic trends will provide the long-term solution to this difficulty – the consultants prefer not to address the problems that arise when these trends turn downwards, as they did in 1990. Meanwhile, the creation – or in some versions recreations – of Enterprise Man (rather less often Woman) in the inner city, individually empowered to address any problems of deprivation that they may encounter, remains the policy objective. An important question that the rhetoric does not help to resolve is whether he or she is an original resident or an incomer.

Such claims are easy to make but difficult to evaluate. The impatience of the House of Commons Public Accounts Committee – basing their criticisms on the National Audit Office evaluation across the broad front of inner city policies (National Audit Office 1990) – with such claims was the trigger for their injunction to the DoE to provide a more systematic and comprehensive evaluation. Unfortunately for us, this will not become available for some time.

Public sector partnerships (the second broad category) embrace a wider range of objectives. In intention at least, they represent an attempt at comprehensive regeneration of the areas concerned, covering economic, environmental and social programmes. It should therefore be possible to apply to them the tests set out in Chapter 3 – essentially, by providing a social profile of the area before and after intervention. Although there are familiar problems of establishing cause and effect and of isolating local, city-wide and regional developments, the analytical difficulties here are largely technical (relating to such questions as the timing of the Census) rather than conceptual. The local inhabitants are essentially conceived of as citizen-tax payers and the issues are around whether they receive fair treatment and value for money in terms of the ability of the public services, suitably enhanced, strengthened, extended or diversified as appropriate, to respond effectively to their needs.

The third approach – popular planning – is a hybrid. In part, it represents a continuation and extension of the local authority-led approach, representing as it does democratic legitimacy (in opposition to the managerial model of the UDC). In its positive mode, it picks up themes of empowerment first evolved by the CDP teams, but in contradistinction to their arguments seeks to apply them to localities rather than on the broader national (or even regional) scene. The policy objective here is to promote direct public involvement in the process of determining the form in which areas should be regenerated and who should share in the benefits of the process. One important measure of success would therefore be the extent of participation and how far those who do participate take an effective part in decision making.

The detail of how participation is achieved raises a series of contestable issues: who is responsible for initiation of action; the role of professionals and those activists who 'parachute' into areas in search of opportunities for effective action; the fate of minorities of all kinds and 'non-joiners'?

Moreover, in order to be successful, a framework has to be set, resources provided and technical skills made available – this inevitably involves some dilution of the 'bottom-up' principle. While it is feasible to evaluate schemes of this kind according to criteria similar to those adopted for the second group, the dimension of community participation will mean that judgements about achievement of goals (or failure to achieve them) may have to be tempered by consideration of the means adopted to reach them.

Some specific criteria

Considering the various forms of deprivation that could be addressed, all the *enterprise strategy* programmes – essentially, the development-led activities of the UDCs – have at some stage set targets for jobs to be generated. Performance under this head has been more fully evaluated in Chapter 9. For present purposes there is a narrower question: how far do the UDCs consider the promotion of training schemes and links between schools and employers as part of their responsibilities? And are other agencies (principally developers) prepared to take a share of the responsibility for provision of such schemes?

In Docklands, the answers to these questions have varied over time. After severe criticism in 1987/8 (see Chapter 6 for details) some share of responsibility for training (in liaison with other agencies) is now accepted by the corporation; and work on school-work links has been instituted. Direct support for two local educational institutions (Tower Hamlets post-16 College, in Poplar, and Bacons City Technology College) now features in the strategic plan. But essentially the process is still market-led. Developers are prepared to enter agreements to employ a proportion of local labour in the construction phase and subsequently. The Tower Hamlets Accord involving Olympia & York's Canary Wharf scheme and Rosehaugh Stanhope's proposals for Royal Docks which led to the Newham Agreement contained detailed provisions on training and education and the use of local labour. But all this activity is relatively marginal, even compared with the numbers of jobs being created.

In the case of other UDCs, there is now a general acceptance of the principle that some provision to enhance employment opportunities for locals is necessary (see for example the memoranda to House of Commons Employment Committee from Merseyside, Teesside, Black Country, Tyne and Wear, Cardiff Bay and Trafford Park DCs (House of Commons Employment Committee 1988b)). This holds true even in cases like Trafford Park, where there is no significant local resident population, although the scale of the training operation supported is, as we have seen, very small. Merseyside DC's programme is considerably larger; 7,100 training places were supported in 1988 – which compares favourably with LDDC at this stage in the evolution of its operations. Black Country DC, despite their Vice-Chair's perception of the limits on their 'tasking', referred in their glossy brochure (which included quotations from Hegel, Herbert Spencer and Delacroix among the colour photographs) to their concern for improving standards of training so that 'young people should be educationally equipped to meet the challenges and opportunities of a regenerated Black country' (Black Country Development Corporation 1989). Devices employed include skills audits, compacts involving local schools and consideration of agreements about the proportion of local labour on new construction schemes. However, there is a problem here (referred to in more detail in Chapter 9) about the legal status of local preference agreements; Olympia & York's ingenious solution is to offer payment of a 'fine' into the community trust. The Centre for Local Economic Strategies comment in their interim appraisal that

> though most local authorities are now making demands on the UDCs about employment and equal opportunity issues they are often not as rigorous or forcefully made as one might expect. Few authorities have set down in writing to the UDC what they expect in terms of jobs, targeting, training or protecting of existing jobs.
>
> (Centre for Local Economic Strategies 1989)

In the case of *public-sector-led* organisations, this difficulty does not arise. Others do. Heartlands is employing much the same set of devices as the UDCs: a skills audit (the results of which are very depressing); an education compact; schemes designed to promote training; special initiatives for women (reflecting the high proportion of house-bound younger single parents in the area); and special projects directed towards the specific needs of ethnic minorities. Important though the emphasis is, much of the running on these issues has been made by the DTI's East Birmingham task force.

The 'public-public' leverage achieved by the task forces is one of their most important contributions and much of this has been applied in local interests – as in the case of schemes targeted towards ethnic minority businesses by the short-lived Handsworth Task Force (PA/Cambridge Economic Consultants 1989). But there is a question about how far the amount of activity they have stimulated survives them – the very short lifespan, intended to promote flexibility, may have the drawback of leaving 'orphan' projects – as seems to have been the case in Handsworth, where the March 1991 appraisal is critical of an inadequately prepared 'exit strategy' (PA/Cambridge Economic Consultants 1991b).

Popular planning does not have many achievements to measure against these; although Labour local authorities (especially the GLC) spent much time on trying to save jobs and generate new activity this was under a different auspice: the promotion of general economic development strategies (Mackintosh and Wainwright 1987). Eventually (where they survived) these initiatives became absorbed into the mainstream of local government activity and adopted many of the entrepreneurial characteristics (as enterprise boards). The local community-generated schemes, of which Coin Street is the most significant example, have not had very significant employment consequences: the emphasis in the commercial part of that development on small workshops is distinctive though not necessarily likely to promote local employment (Brindley *et al.* 1989: 88). But the people's plan for Royal Docks in East London (prepared with support from the GLC) is of interest, mainly for its attempt to base an alternative approach on revival of employment in the docks themselves (thereby attempting to protect traditional docklands occupations rather than attempting to innovate (see Brownill 1990: 128)).

Housing is an altogether different matter. UDCs are not housing authorities. However, those that contain substantial residential areas have been drawn willy-nilly into the issue of provision of housing – both how it should be provided and the form that it should take – and the rehabilitation of existing dwellings (which do, after all, form part of the built environment). LDDC is again the paradigm case. By encouraging speculative private sector housing development LDDC has achieved a substantial increase in the numbers of dwellings and almost equally spectacular turn-round in the tenure mix. Is this success? In terms of homes for locals, clearly not; the new housing has been predominantly built for sale at prices that local people cannot possibly afford; attempts to provide affordable housing were a fiasco and the boroughs cannot build for rent – the DC has taken most of their housing land and their HIPs have been severely cut. Housing associations have also suffered from constraints on public spending and from the provision in the 1988 Housing Act that limits Housing Association Grant to 75 per cent of the cost of developments (see Chapter 6 for detailed evidence).

In terms of ministerial objectives, however, the changes in Docklands are clearly a move in the right direction. Commenting on building for sale in Docklands, Michael Heseltine observes, 'at last the successful were being courted, not driven away'. The process (he claims) reflected the importance of rebuilding 'balanced, socially mixed communities'; Heseltine's illustration of new private construction is captioned 'Only the Left protest' (Heseltine 1987, facing p. 153). This, however, is not the case; and LDDC's enforced retreat on the social housing issue in the face of sustained criticism from all quarters (see Chapter 6) is one of the most interesting of several changes of direction after 1987. The difficulty about implementation of the agreements that LDDC has now reached with Newham and Tower Hamlets (trading planning permission for new rented homes) is that they require very substantial injections of public money through the DoE's funding allocation to Docklands. The problem here is that the DoE has until now not been anxious to divert funds in this direction – and the mishandling of the transport infrastructure means that there are other imperative calls on resources if LDDC is to retain its credibility as a redevelopment agency.

Other UDCs have not been faced with the same problem. The CLES interim appraisal comments that while new private housing – especially in waterfront sites – has acted as a lead sector for some UDCs (notably Cardiff Bay): 'the main issue for most authorities in the declining industrial regions is employment rather than housing so new housing developments attract less adverse comment' (Centre for Local Economic Strategies 1989: 19). Trafford Park DC, with no significant resident population, has kept out of the housing field altogether, with the exception of a marginal involvement in canal-side private development by the Manchester Ship Canal Company (see Chapter 5).

Housing was also initially 'a low-key issue' for Merseyside DC (Dawson and Parkinson 1991: 53). But the enlargement of the Development Corporation's boundaries in 1988 brought the question of affordable housing to the centre of debate – one in which the MDC was clearly anxious to avoid stepping into the same minefield as LDDC. Enlargement has also brought MDC into a working relationship with one of the largest new build housing cooperatives in the country, the Eldonian Community in Vauxhall. In these circumstances, Merseyside DC, 'concerned to develop a cooperative rather than a confrontational stance', developed a partnership approach through the formulation of area strategies with substantial participation both by local people and the local authorities. However, a potential problem for Merseyside – as for some other corporations – is that any successes in achieving physical rehabilitation through community-led schemes and improvement of the local environment may, through stimulating developer interest, squeeze out further social housing in favour of more profitable commercial development (Dawson and Parkinson 1991: 55).

The relative strengths of the collaborative public partnerships (Heartlands and GEAR) lie in avoiding the problems faced by UDCs with significant residential populations: turning the problem over to the private sector and opting out of social housing altogether with the exception of a strictly limited role for housing associations (which can be passed off as part of the 'enterprise sector') inevitably produces criticisms of lack of substantial benefit for locals. Heartlands' housing programme is balanced between a relatively modest programme of new development (led by developers: Bordesley Village) and a substantial public sector demolition/ rehabilitation programme led by the City Housing Department (Nechells), with some significant tenant input (Bloomsbury Estate Management Board). Changes that visibly benefit locals are therefore included in the programme from the outset. A similar pattern emerged in east Glasgow in GEAR, with SDA playing the same role as the developers in the Heartlands consortium. In both cases, the old-style public sector paternalism has not altogether been avoided; but Colin Ward, revisiting Glasgow after a long interval, found the environment 'dramatically' improved (Ward 1989: 49). If the pace of change in these schemes is not always as rapid as it might be, Stockbridge Village Trust provides a salutary warning of what can occur if highly deprived housing estates are handed over without proper safeguards to a private sector-led operation – even in the guise of a non-profit trust (see p. 224 above).

Within the very limited group of popular planning initiatives, Coin Street stands out as providing a potential alternative, with its intensive use of community-based housing associations as the means for providing adequate housing in a location and form explicitly intended to match community needs. Although the quantity of housing provided will not be great, the participative model can be seen to have achieved significant results here. The inner city can also now show some evidence of the viability of the most participative model of all – self-build housing on the Isle of Dogs (for which see Ward 1989: 53).

So it seems clear that in this area at least the development-led model of UDC, with its vulnerability to recession and particularly dependence on the notoriously volatile housing market (especially in the south east), has less to offer than a balanced approach employing resources of both public and private sector – and involving housing associations. That is, unless the real goal is taken to be achieving political change through changing population structure, as Michael Heseltine's comments have sometimes seemed to imply.

Environment and image

Much of the debate around urban policy in the course of the 1980s has been directed towards the question of reversing the negative image of inner city areas and thereby instigating their revival not just as centres of economic activity but as places to live. Here, at least, the objectives of economic and social policy may connect. One of the keys to revival that has been built into many of the enterprise-led schemes has been environmental improvement, seen in its most flamboyant form in the garden festivals that spread across the inner cities of Britain over the 1980s like a green rash.

Much of this type of activity can be categorised alongside the logo and the glossy brochures (with past photographed in black-and-white and present in full colour) as part of the hype designed to impress potential investors. Hence it has no place in this analysis (see Chapter 9). However, it should be added that a consultant's report for the DoE (PA/Cambridge Economic Consultants) on the garden festivals reports that if the cost of derelict land grant (which would, it is argued, have to be expended whether festivals had been held or not) is disregarded, festivals 'deliver similar, if not better results than other projects used in inner city regeneration' (*Independent*, 20 October 1990).

But other efforts at improvement of the environment are directed not outwards to possible developers but inwards to the existing inhabitants. A not entirely predictable characteristic of consultations with local people is that they have repeatedly thrown up demands for more public open space (in Heartlands, for one) and for leisure facilities of decent standard. City Farms, a new development in the early 1970s, has spread 'not through any official body but from local enthusiasm' (Ward 1989: 100); one of the best known is at the Mudchute, in Docklands.

Such facilities, of course, are not only attractive from the point of view of existing residents; developers have also used them as incentives for attracting new purchasers to their new private-sector housing developments, as employers do to entice new members of staff. Or they have been provided as a part of 'planning gain' deals – petty ransom for proceeding with large-scale developments. In Stockbridge a 'Caribbean-style' leisure centre was seen as one of the keys to turning the derelict tower blocks of the estate into flats suitable for young middle-class couples. In Heartlands the (draft) social strategy bristles with proposals for upgrading existing libraries and community centres as a new focus for the area. Either way, the provision of high quality leisure services (community or development based) can be read as symbols of the willingness of the agencies responsible to invest in the future of the neighbourhood. Sustaining them can in turn be seen as an index of restored morale, especially where they are managed by the community as well as in the neighbourhood.

The focus for social action

But this approach poses a difficulty: what exactly does the term 'neighbourhood' imply? As we have already pointed out in the course of the case-studies, almost all the UDCs (and both Heartlands and GEAR) are based on geographical units that are essentially artificial. Attempts made to give them a real existence may cut against one of the existing community's few assets: their positive identification with the locality with which they are familiar and desire to see it improved. This clinging to the 'real' neighbourhood, rather than the imposed new description, turns up repeatedly in social surveys, so the use of distinctive logos, public display of symbols, 'flagship' developments with cute titles and the building of 'gateways' to areas may be positively counter-productive – still more so, the higher nonsense of seeking 'sexy' titles to rechristen those areas judged to be too severely affected to be redeemed under their original name (thus Cantril Farm became Stockbridge Village). These attempts to create a coherent identity where none has previously existed in areas defined in terms of their potential for physical regeneration – while they may sometimes be valid as the focus for economically-focused action – perfectly epitomise the disjunction between social and economic objectives that has characterised urban policy, both public and private sector led, since the 1977 White Paper.

CDPs sought to heal the breach by abandoning any serious attempt at area-based action and concentrating on the overarching structural issues. Their successors in the 1980s have reverted to the small area approach as a way (by analogy with much-admired Third World resistance movements) of liberating a few square miles of territory where an attempt can be made to demonstrate how things might be better done. Within this territory – in the 'locality' (preferred term) – the issues that have been evolved by the 'rainbow coalition' of interests within the new model Labour party can be pursued as a matter of first priority until the inevitable day dawns when the forces of the central state prove too powerful, thereby satisfying the final requirement in the psychodrama of 'struggle'. And many of these issues are essentially social policy questions: improved child care facilities; women's centres with crèches; improved training facilities specifically targeted at minorities; equal opportunities policies. That these (and other) issues should find themselves on the inner city agenda is clearly right; their brusque sidelining as part of the early 1980s physical regeneration-at-all-costs strategy has already been shown to be shortsighted. Nor is there much dispute about the need for the public sector to take a lead in ensuring that these issues are attended to: private sector interest is too capricious and ephemeral. These areas fall outside the areas of concern – and indeed competence – of all but those rare firms that have a systematic social responsibility programme: though those that have both have made a significant impact.

But if the public sector is to take a lead on a range of social issues, it does not follow from experience so far that it must necessarily itself take responsibility for the delivery of services. This opens up the other main question. If the outcome of private sector-led (or private–public) initiatives is that local residents do not obtain access to good quality social facilities or are not equipped with the financial means to purchase them elsewhere, are there other methods – community-based self-help or other forms of voluntary action, for example – that will help to provide them?

Community involvement

Backwash from the CDP episode helped to discredit any notion that government – central or local – should be directly involved in promoting community development. But another lesson was also learned: new developments have to carry people with them, because the consequence of failing to do so may attract the kind of publicity that compromises the success of operation. It is a common characteristic of all three major types of development being described that public consultation has been built in. But it takes different forms and is provided to meet different objectives.

With the UDCs the chosen means have been glossy publications backed by leafleting and telephone hot lines. Latterly, some development corporations have held public meetings and open forum discussions, and occasionally conducted surveys of opinion. This approach appears to be based on the notion that consultation will somehow add to the authenticity of decisions taken – hence the farce of Trafford Park DC reporting community consultation as the rationale for a traffic scheme when there is actually no resident community. More often, the approach is through informal discussions with carefully selected groups with particular interests that impinge on those of the corporation.

But at the same time, it is seen as essential not to compromise the commercial advantage to be gained from the UDCs' 'apolitical' status as single-purpose authorities by permitting lengthy debate on proposals – so at the outset London Docklands DC imposed a fourteen-day limit on consultation and held no inquiries (see Chapter 6). The natural response of well-established local groups was to dig their heels in: some (minor) victories were gained but even (relatively) well-heeled Docklands groups found it difficult to make any substantial progress except through confrontational tactics. However, successful manipulation of media through high-profile events (the release of the unfortunate sheep from Mudchute City Farm into a formal meeting; the Docklands Armada of small boats sailing down river to Westminster) achieved some impact, through inflicting damage on the LDDC's image.

The LDDC's response to pressure has been threefold: initially, to suggest that the groups concerned were not genuinely representative of the community; then to stress that the need for rapid action was of paramount importance (so locals should 'share the vision' rather than carp); and then to increase their use of consultants as surrogate for consultation. But eventually LDDC abandoned this negative position and started taking the need to carry locals with them seriously. The Community Services Division was set up, outreach workers were hired, Planning Committee meetings were opened and more consultative meetings held ('don't slip on the soft soap', said one activist to another at the door).

A redesigned approach of this kind, if promoted with sophistication and commitment, poses a real dilemma for community groups. It requires them to combine a range of functions that may not be compatible (can they be representative, advocacy and protest organisations all at once?). How do existing voluntary bodies and groups representing special interests (ethnic minorities, disability groups) fit into the picture? Some of them (the churches and other religious groups) may have genuine local roots; but others may simply be hastily created as vehicles for bodies active on a wider scene – the national level, even – who see the area as a possible location for new activities (and grants). What role do organisations based around the workplace – trades unions, in particular – have to play? In what sense do all these local activities coalesce to form a 'community' (a term of which all fight shy these days)?

And at the end of it all, what long-term benefit can local people realistically expect for themselves? The famous victory over the developers at Covent Garden in the 1970s is often held out as an example of people power in action; but when the dust settled the local working class were not among the main beneficiaries (Anson 1981); the voices that spoke most effectively were those of the middle-class professionals and, welcome though the area's survival with its buildings largely intact may be, it serves largely as a playground for young professional people.

It is fair to add that LDDC is not at all typical; the growth or in some cases implantation of groups in Docklands took place long before the development corporation was declared and was nourished by support from the GLC (Mackintosh and Wainwright 1987). In other UDCs there is a much smaller and less self-consciously oppositional population – where there has been a population at all.

There is a key contrast here with the public-sector-led regeneration schemes in Heartlands and Glasgow East End. GEAR and, until recent changes, Heartlands UDA, retained full functional local authority linkages, and lines of accountability still exist; and though the style is paternalistic the structure is familiar and to some extent accessible. The traditional political structures survive and, if necessary, can be invoked.

Active attempts at further involvement of local people have been made in both cases (see Chapter 6 and Donnison and Middleton 1987). Although the initial consultation in Heartlands was generally agreed to have been a fiasco, local opposition fizzled out after some early gestures and involvement in specific housing schemes was relatively successful. Most groups are artificial creations in the sense that they exist in the context of specific local government activities – hence Birmingham Housing Department's references to 'our' tenants' associations.

The vacuum that exists as a result leaves space for a role for the existing voluntary sector and churches and other non-Christian religious bodies. Their representational and advocacy role can be very important in keeping alternative channels open – which are needed despite the continued existence of the political structures. Archbishops may, as we suggested earlier, be prone to become excitable about trickle down and the limits on its effectiveness; but they have also been prepared to put the Church's money where their mouth has been. The Churches' urban fund, established in 1988, represents in some senses a return to the Church of England's traditional concerns with inner poverty in 'Darkest England' but cased in a new form, with its stress on community projects and with an ecumenical flavour.

Finally, in the third category of activity, popular planning, the people are part of the process so that issues around the form and nature of participation shouldn't be crucial. But are they? Are women fully involved? Are black people? Brownill's account of the Docklands experience suggests that eternal vigilance is needed if tokenism in representation (to take only one central issue) is to be avoided (Brownill 1990).

All these alternative strategies are superfluous – or at best mere froth on the surface – if the policy objective remains economic regeneration first and last and the beneficiaries are to be the entrepreneurs about their hustle and bustle and (at a decent remove) the enterprising and empowered. But a concern with participation and partnership becomes an essential ingredient once it is accepted that policy can have other, broader objectives and that the beneficiaries should include those who have experienced the deprivations.

11 Private investment as public policy

Before we go on to draw our final conclusions there is one further point that should be made: put simply, it is that there is nothing really new in the enterprise-based approach to inner city regeneration. Despite the sugar coating of rhetoric and the various presentational 'spins' that have been applied from time to time, much of what has been attempted is visibly familiar – and to that extent the outcome has been predictable. The use of the private sector of the economy for the promotion and pursuit of public ends has a long, if not very distinguished history. The 1934 Special Areas Act provided powers for 'the initiation, organisation, prosecution and assistance of measures to facilitate the economic development and social improvement' of the special areas (otherwise known as the depressed areas) (see Cullingworth 1985: 7–8). This included the provision and improvement of services, amenity schemes and the clearing of derelict sites. But as Cullingworth notes, all this was to be complementary to the principal task of attracting new industry to the depressed areas. Apart from the use of specially designated corporations therefore, there is little difference between the aims of the 1934 Act and the purpose of current inner city policy. And the lessons from inter-war policy seem only too familiar. Attempts to exploit the social responsibility and community-mindedness of industry singularly failed. Only where inducements (in the form of the provision of trading estates) were offered did industry respond. But even then three times as many factories opened in the London area as in all the special areas combined between 1937 and 1938.

With the benefit of longer-term hindsight, subsequent history proved to be only a little more effective. Fifty years after the Barlow Report (Barlow Report 1940) which had its origins in depressed area policies, the experience of enticing and cajoling industry into doing something it probably would not otherwise have done is less than encouraging – at least in any terms other than simple physical relocation. The industrial location policies of the 1960s were aimed (as are current UDC policies) at reducing unemployment, though in much larger areas (the development areas) but did not markedly change the relative regional distribution of unemployment and disadvantage (see Fothergill and Gudgin 1982; Balchin and Bull 1987). Again, the Assisted Areas Scheme under the Industry Act 1972 attempted (with a modicum of success) to lure industry into designated areas with the use of subsidies and other inducements, but if the purpose was to transform the assisted areas into the growth loci of enterprise, the results are a long time coming.

The most direct of the forebears of the urban development corporations were of course the new town development corporations upon which they are in part modelled. Indeed, the wording of parts of the two acts that brought these quangos into existence (the New Towns Act 1965 and the Local Government Planning and Land Act 1980) is identical. However, to search for the provenance of success in the experience of the new towns would be misguided. Institutionally the new town story can be said to have been a success (see Aldridge 1979; Schaffer 1972), but there the similarity ends. Superficially, at least, the purposes of the two types of development corporation pull in opposite directions – one *out* of the cities, the other into them. And the job that the urban development corporations have to do (in relieving urban deprivation) is altogether more complex. The relative success of the new towns therefore (on *some* indicators, at least) provides little or no 'form' to assess the performance of the inner city corporations.

It is worth noting briefly some of the essential characteristics of these attempts (which, methodologically, from the special areas schemes of the 1930s to the urban development corporations of the 1990s are all very similar) to bend the activities of the private sector in the service of public goals. The first point to note is that these attempts must be distinguished from the much broader area of government intervention in the private sector for the purposes of controlling or regulating or policing private sector activity and its consequences. Bending private sector activity in the manner we are describing is quite unlike the control exercised in the maintenance of health and safety or the policing of pollution or any other regulatory measure (including the negative side of industrial location policy such as the industrial development certificates in operation during the 1970s).

The second feature that characterises the policies that we have identified is that all use inducements of one sort or another to bend private sector activity. Indeed, when regulation and control are excluded as policy instruments, there is little left to governments by way of 'behaviour modification techniques' other than a variety of carrots. In this respect therefore, current inner city policy differs only in detail from special area policies of sixty years ago. The succulence of the carrots of course is a matter of judgement and it was, as we have noted, a matter of concern to the Treasury that, so far as the UDCs were concerned, they would have to be too big and juicy. The ultimate test, however, would be the gearing ratio. But at least the Treasury recognised that the enterprise strategy was not going to be costless.

Thirdly, as we have noted elsewhere, a necessary concomitant of the logistics of enticement is area designation. What distinguishes inner city policy from its forebears in this regard is of course the size of the areas designated. Urban development areas are, to all intents and purposes, industrial location policy writ small.

But the difference in size may also entail a difference in the quality of the outcome. The smaller the area designated for enticement, the more arbitrary and extraordinary it is likely to be. There should, after all, be very special reasons for wanting to designate a few thousand acres of land (and often less) as opposed to a region or part of a region. It implies some special significance for the area and for the consequences of regenerating it. And that special significance, as we have seen, is usually attributed to something called an inner city economy.

A fourth feature common to most manipulated industrial location is that if it is to work on any scale, recipient areas cannot afford to be too choosy about what types of industry or other economic activity relocate (or locate) there. Certainly, so far as the UDCs are concerned, most have preferences (often for particular sites) but at the end of the day, the pressures of the gearing ratio will dictate a more opportunistic attitude to incoming economic activity. The immediate consequence of this is that any fine-tuning of the types of jobs that are created (or relocated) is virtually impossible. There is little possibility of fitting the profile of new jobs – that is, assuming that they do not arrive complete with incumbents – to the mix of skills to be found in the local (unemployed) labour force. Any 'fitting' has to be in the reverse direction: the local unemployed must be trained up to fit whatever profile of jobs results from the enticement.

Finally, inducements do not operate in a vacuum; they are one of many considerations of which companies will take account when deciding where to locate, relocate, expand and so on, or indeed, whether to do so. But of greatest importance is the fact that location, start-up and expansion decisions will be subject to the economic climate and this has been all too evident in the recent experience of the urban development corporations, as our case-studies have shown. Investment decisions will always be subject to economic cycles and in times of recession such inducements as are on offer by urban development corporations or related bodies will probably provide scant incentive. In this, of course, current inner city policy does not differ from its predecessors: to hitch public policy to the fortunes of the private sector is to make it subject to the vicissitudes of the economy in a very direct way.

EVALUATING THE ENTERPRISE STRATEGY

Like the industrial location policies of the 1960s and 1970s therefore, the main benefits of the enterprise strategy for the inner city should be from targeted job creation. But there are two important respects (as well as a number of lesser ones) in which inner city policy differs from earlier industrial location strategies. The first is a direct consequence of the size of the designated areas. Whilst it is no less likely that migrant firms to special or assisted areas will bring at least some of their work-force with them, hence reducing the opportunities for the local work-force, they are more likely, when they *do* recruit, to take on people from the designated area simply by virtue of its size. When the designated area and its labour force hinterland are that much smaller however (as with inner city designations) there is a far greater likelihood that employees will be drawn from beyond the inner cities, thus further reducing the opportunities for local benefit. Secondly, the *intended* consequences of the enterprise strategy go far beyond just job creation. It has been our purpose in preceding chapters to elaborate on the job that the enterprise strategy is meant to do, and we need not cover that ground again here. Suffice it to say that the (relatively) simple output of new job creation (allied to skills training) is required, through the medium of trickle down, confidence-building and the rejuvenation of inner city economies, to make substantial inroads into urban deprivation in its many manifestations. This is considerably more than the special areas and assisted areas schemes were ever meant to achieve.

Now it will be argued in defence of government policy, as we have noted in earlier chapters, that the enterprise strategy was never intended to be the entirety of inner city policy. The Urban Programme, it will be argued, stands as strong testimony to that. Such a counter would be true in a literal sense but it has been our contention that presentationally and financially, governments over the past ten years *have* put most of their eggs in the enterprise basket and continue to do so. The distribution of funds within the urban block and the priority given to urban development corporations makes that point perfectly clear. What is really at issue therefore is how much the enterprise strategy can achieve – in theory and in practice – and how much of that congeries of problems we call urban deprivation will only be susceptible to other measures including, and most importantly, service provision. As a prerequisite therefore of a consideration of what else is needed, we shall rehearse the limitations of the enterprise strategy both as a matter of social logic and as the evidence from our case-studies dictates.

Too much has been claimed for the enterprise approach and it will not be long before the government is disowning the hyperbole of the glossy brochures just as chairmen and chief executives of some urban development corporations are already doing. They contain too many hostages to fortune as well as sounding increasingly silly (by which we mean singularly unconvincing). Job creation is an essential part of any strategy to alleviate urban deprivation but its potential for generating further change must be kept in perspective. In the logic of the enterprise culture, the inner city economy was to be a key instrument in regeneration, but we have found no evidence of the existence of such (even relatively) discrete entities either in our case-study areas or elsewhere. It certainly stretches credulity to think of the large international financial institutions that were, in more buoyant times, clamouring to get into London Docklands as part of an inner city economy. Inner city economies owe more to a combination of mercantile fantasy and craft-workshop optimism than to anything that resembles a realistic assessment of present day economic exigencies. And if we are to match 'brochure-talk' with reality, it is hard to reconcile the monumental (in both its senses) towers of Docklands or Trafford Park or Merseyside Docklands with 'hustle and bustle on a human scale'.

The enterprise strategy has also relied heavily, in logistical terms, on the notion of spatially definable and discrete inner cities and this also we have found wanting in a number of respects. If by inner city areas we mean areas of relative concentration of various mixes of components of urban deprivation, then the evidence is clear that such concentrations do not occur in neatly described areas. There is great heterogeneity in inner city areas: different types of deprivation are often widely scattered; neighbourhoods may be identified by their residents by only one or two blocks of houses, and pockets of deprivation may exist cheek-by-jowl with areas of relative affluence. In short, the inner cities are not the spatially definable homogeneous entities that the logic of enterprise regeneration requires. The implication of this is that attempts to regenerate *the* inner city economy or *the* inner city will fail and they will fail because they are predicated on assumptions about the nature of the inner city which are fundamentally flawed. It is from such assumptions for example that flow the beliefs that investment needs to be located in the inner city to be of benefit to it, and that area designations as policy instruments bear some meaningful relation to concentrations of deprivation. None of these assumptions survives scrutiny, as the examples of Heartlands, LDDC and TPDC have shown.

If the enterprise strategy is fundamentally flawed however, this does not mean that elements of it are not valuable. Stripped of its ideological veneer and more extravagant claims, one of its central elements – job creation – must remain as a necessary component of any inner city strategy. But how it might be accomplished and what it might achieve require reassessment. If it is accepted that job creation is all that needs to be salvaged from the enterprise strategy and that any ideas of regenerating discrete inner cities and inner city economies can be sloughed off, then the mechanics of how this can be achieved need to be redesigned. Firstly, the logistics of entice-ment will have to remain in place and this must include some form of area designation. Stripped to its essentials, what is required is more jobs that are accessible to (that is, within a reasonable distance of work) the main concentrations of unemployed people in cities, combined with the provision of suitable training and skills development. This means that subsidies of one sort or another must remain in place to optimise the possibilities of attracting new investment. It also means that areas must continue to be defined within which the subsidies operate and outwith which they do not. Until better and more effective means of enticement can be found therefore (and after sixty years of operation, none has), 'subsidies-with-designations' will have to remain, and, with them, their two main dysfunctions – negative extra-boundary effects and susceptibility to economic change – along with several subsidiary dysfunctions including limitations on the control of what types of job are generated and the fact that training and skills provision always seem (at least on past experience) to be optional add-ons to policy. Within these limitations however, job creation can be pursued in a more realistic manner than that adopted in the enterprise strategy.

The designated areas need not pretend to describe regenerative economies or inner city areas. Given the essential requirement identified above, these areas need be no more than loci for business, commercial and industrial expansion and location, within travel-to-work distance of con-centrations of unemployed people. Rather than discrete economies, they might best be thought of as business commercial and industrial 'parks'. There is of course nothing new in this and indeed, Trafford Park provides us with an obvious model. The strategy is therefore a simpler one and pretends to nothing more than job creation where it is of use to people who need it. Perhaps its main distinctive feature however is that it has no ambitions of the 'hustle and bustle on a human scale' variety, seeking only to establish concentrations of employment physically separated wherever possible and desirable from residential areas. There may well be circum-stances of course where local populations might on balance want, or prefer, some mixed use in their areas. This would seem to be most obviously a case for local consultation and participation but in all likelihood it will depend on the nature and size of the new investment. It has been our contention that new employment on the scale necessary to have any significant impact on local unemployment rates will not be achieved only or mainly by small establishments such as shops, workshops or studio factories, but will require some large-scale enterprises. It is less likely that the location of these in, or proximate to, residential areas would prove to be acceptable.

Perhaps the most sensitive aspect of such an employment strategy would be the location of the 'investment parks'. We have said that their obvious location must be within travel-to-work distance of concentrations of unemployed people. This would be the optimum solution, but there will no doubt be instances where suitable and available sites do not exist within reasonable travel distances of inner city areas with large numbers of unemployed people. In such cases some alternative to the 'investment park' solution would have to be found. Whatever else inner city policy has taught us over the past decade, we should have learned that no single strategy will fit all of the wide variety of inner city problems.

A more intractable difficulty, and one that may in part define the limits of effectiveness of the simple employment-strategy (just as it does of the more ambitious enterprise strategy), is that geographic concentrations of unemployed people may not (and on the ecological evidence we have cited earlier, often will not) coincide with concentrations of people suffering from a variety of other components of deprivation. The *apparent* consequence of this is that the relative absence of ecological contiguity of unemployment and other deprivations will limit any potential trickle down effect there may have been from job creation. In reality, however, as we have noted previously, apart from any (and usually minor) environmental effects, the trickle down process is not an ecological one but more likely (or more often) an intra-family, or intra-household one, and to this extent the lack of spatial coincidence of deprivations is probably irrelevant. The limit of trickle down from job creation is not therefore a spatial one since trickle down does not operate spatially. (Of course, where spatial contiguity results from the coincidence within families or households of unemployment and other deprivations, the ecological dimension may be said to disappear.)

In general therefore, we must say that the *operational* limits of the employment strategy (as opposed to such factors as susceptibility to the economic climate) are twofold and both are shared with the enterprise strategy. The first is that there is no empirical evidence that trickle down has anything other than a minor effect. Certainly, there is nothing to suggest that it is an effective mechanism for relieving dependency on a large scale. The second is that because trickle down operates at the household or family level, its spatial effects are an accidental by-product of the intra-household coincidence of deprivations.

Employment growth will therefore have only marginal effects on deprivations in areas with low unemployment rates or where there are few people in the labour market. In these areas, and for those components of deprivation that trickle down does not reach, quite different strategies will have to be adopted.

So much then for the process and limits of a 'simple' job creation strategy. But what of other elements of the enterprise strategy and in particular, the organisation and institutional elements? Should they remain in place, or can they be jettisoned along with the strategy's less realistic ambitions?

It will be recalled that the enterprise strategy was fuelled, particularly in the mid-1980s, by a strong distrust of local authorities on the part of government. If the strategy were to thrive therefore, new agencies would have to be created which would pursue it single-mindedly. Would these agencies still be needed to effect the simpler job creation strategy we have outlined, and what alternatives, if any, present themselves? There are two fronts on which to approach this question. The first is what sorts of agencies are best able to attract investment and create jobs. The second is, what sorts of agencies are most likely to be able to extract local benefit from new investment. Only the first is directly related to the job creation strategy as such, but the second must also be a relevant consideration.

In previous chapters, we have looked at three types of 'agency arrangement' in the loose sense of that term: urban development corporations, a 'pure private' arrangement (really a non-agency) and a local authority – private sector partnership. A fourth arrangement would of course be local authorities acting alone. The track record of UDCs to date on job creation is a mixed one so far as it is possible to judge from official figures that appear consistently to be laundered. Certainly some of the more exotic figures quoted by the LDDC bear little relation to more reasoned estimates. Trafford Park Development Corporation is some 3,000 or so jobs towards its target of 16,000 but that, as we have noted, seems an unduly modest one. The results for other development corporations are so far disappointing. To offset that, however, we have to consider what might have happened had the UDCs not been designated. We know that Trafford Metropolitan Borough invited the designation of TPDC in the belief that this would be the most effective means of achieving the regeneration of Trafford Park, and other authorities have seen UDC designation as a means of getting government resources into their area which they would otherwise not receive. The counter-argument, particularly on the part of the London Boroughs of Tower Hamlets, Southwark and Newham, has been that had they received the levels of resource from which the LDDC has benefited, they could have done the job just as well. That must be viewed with a degree of scepticism, for reasons that we have developed at greater length in Chapter 6.

But the fact is of course that where local authorities had wanted to take action to attract investment to their inner cities, the best expedient was to attract UDC status because, given the ideological fix of the three Conservative governments during the 1980s, there was little chance otherwise of getting the necessary resources. Those that resisted the importation of UDC machinery and the loss of their powers that went with it – as Birmingham did – had to accept that any additional funds would be provided case by case, on a grace and favour basis and not in the form of direct grants. In Birmingham's case, this restriction eventually brought about a change of direction and acceptance of UDC machinery in modified form. The alternative of local authority-led economic regeneration has been effectively foreclosed for more than a decade so that any direct comparisons with development corporation-led regeneration is not possible. That having been said, there is no evidence (unless inaction during the 1970s be taken as such) that local authorities, given the power and the resources, *would* not be as effective at job creation as urban development corporations.

Of the other two 'arrangements', it is too early to judge the effectiveness of Heartlands (the only substantial example to date of the private sector-local authority arrangement) as an instrument for job creation, especially in view of the changes that have now occurred there. The 'pure private' approach exemplified by the Trafford Centre will only ever produce happenstance job growth in so far as – by definition – it will not result from an enticement strategy. It is, however, as earlier chapters have shown, within the power of local authorities, by means of planning consents and trade-offs, to facilitate such development and the net benefits in terms of jobs created can be very considerable. (The Trafford Centre alone would create twice as many jobs as have been produced in the whole of the remainder of the Trafford Park designated area since 1987.) Other things being equal therefore, local authorities would be unwise to eschew the job creation potential of the private sector wherever this could be of benefit to the inner cities.

As to whether special agencies such as urban development corporations are a necessary facilitator of a 'simple' policy of job creation (as opposed to 'inner city regeneration') therefore, we can only veer away from agnosticism on the strength of the lack of any evidence that local authorities, given similar powers and resources, could not do the job as effectively. This of course implies a presumption in favour of local authorities but this seems reasonable on the grounds that there is no point in creating new agencies if it is not necessary. Unless and until it can be shown conclusively therefore that special agencies are more effective and efficient at job creation than are local authorities (and the evidence so far does not point in this direction), there is little point in their further use.

Extracting local benefit is an adjunct to the job creation strategy. It does not imply any reversion to the extravagant claims of the enterprise culture to regenerate inner city economies or revitalise inner city areas. It is simply a matter of ensuring that as many of the new jobs as possible go to unemployed local people. We have already canvassed the means by which this might potentially be done: tailored training programmes, agreements to employ local labour, conditions to planning consents to give preference to the local work-force and so on. Almost all of this activity requires some form of partnership or arrangement between the private sector and whatever agency is responsible for providing training, extracting local benefit and so on. Our second line of approach therefore is whether some agency arrangements are more effective at extracting local benefit than others.

The evidence from our two development corporation case-studies is not impressive. Concern about local benefit came late in the day at LDDC and there is little evidence that job creation in Docklands has produced much benefit for local people. The Trafford Park Development Corporation 'assumes' that many of the 3,000 or so jobs created have gone to local people but has not monitored this and has no firm data. Neither development corporation has entered binding agreements with migrant firms over local labour. These 'single-minded bodies' it would seem have been all too single-minded on their drive for high gearing ratios to the exclusion of any robust efforts to channel growth to benefit local people. Local authorities on the other hand have a more direct interest in promoting local benefit. Their success however (as would be the case with any agency) will depend, as we have noted above, on their ability to arrive at binding agreements with migrant firms. And herein lies the real difficulty with any strategy that relies on cooperation with the private sector.

Making agreements with companies over the employment of local labour, the use of tailored training and setting targets, is one thing; enforcing them is another. Potentially migrant firms may extract all sorts of concessions from local authorities (or other agencies) desperate for the new jobs in return for promises about maximising local benefit, only to renege on such promises when their fulfilment becomes inconvenient or time-consuming. This in fact is just what has happened in the United States on a wide scale (see Barnekov *et al.* 1989, Chapters 5 and 8).

It would seem, therefore, that it probably doesn't much matter what sort of agency is involved in trying to bring benefit to the local population from job creation (let alone economic regeneration) so long as any agreements entered into are unenforceable. There is a possible exception that in a partnership such as existed in Heartlands there may be a somewhat stronger moral commitment to honour agreements, but even there, if companies find the task too onerous, they can, with impunity, simply renege upon them.

We remain pessimistic therefore, in the absence of anything like contract compliance legislation, about the effectiveness of any agency to exploit even the simpler strategy of job creation for the benefit of local unemployed people. This is not to say that efforts and agreements in this direction should not be made – some attempts will no doubt pay off – but it is to recognise the simple truth that the private sector is not in business to bring relief to the urban deprived.

20:20 HINDSIGHT?

So much for the performance of enterprise-based initiatives on their own terms. But there are broader objectives, beyond economic regeneration, that they have from time to time been represented as addressing; and alternative means of satisfying these broader objectives. We refer here to the general attempts to 'do something about those inner cities' (in the former Prime Minister's words) as foci of social deprivation, visible representations of dependency and its consequences and potential locations of violence and social unrest.

Here again, the initial response of the government has been that 'single-minded' agencies have a clear advantage in addressing these problems, in part because they are able to act decisively outwith traditional bureaucratic constraints and in part because they are better able to forge effective working relationships with the private sector and (it has latterly been argued) with inner city communities. This conclusion has been applied both to UDCs and to the inner city task forces, whose role has been seen as providing direct assistance in a form which will immediately benefit inner city inhabitants, particularly those who want to shed their dependent status and try to improve their own circumstances through self-help. The archetypes of these 'deserving' residents would be young blacks attempting to start their own businesses and task forces (especially the one in Handsworth) have made a particular point of trying to meet these needs.

The government's critics point to a number of deficiencies that they perceive in this approach. In general terms the efforts of UDCs are seen as marginal and spasmodic, without long-term commitment. The fact that the existence of UDCs is time-limited often seems to be overlooked; and while the changes that they can achieve in the physical environment may be lasting (alas!), their social schemes are often by their nature limited in scope and ephemeral in their consequences (see Chapter 10). If this is true of the activities of UDCs, it is likely to be more so in the case of task forces. The inability to sustain progress made in helping local black groups in Handsworth is a key example, to which reference has already been made. In both cases, the importance of devising an effective 'exit strategy' has been stressed in consultants' and other evaluations (PA/Cambridge Economic Consultants 1991a and b).

But was the entry of these 'single-purpose' agencies to this field justified in the first place? We would propose three themes against which the relevance of the enterprise strategy and alternative approaches could be measured: accountability, empowerment and partnership.

The absence of effective means of securing accountability has been one of the main criticisms levelled against UDCs from the outset (see House of Commons Employment Committee 1988b; London Docklands Consultative Committee 1987, 1991; Centre for Local Economic Strategies 1989; Colenutt 1991; Dawson and Parkinson 1991, and analysis in Chapter 10). While economic benefits appeared to be flowing freely in the mid- and late-1980s these criticisms fell on deaf ears; but since 1988 there has been a change of emphasis, most notably in the Docklands case where there is now much talk of being responsive to community needs. Without being excessively cynical, the explanation for this change of direction can be located in the economic recession and the impossibility of continuing to assert that benefits would *inevitably* flow from single-minded pursuit of physical regeneration policies. Whether the new face of Docklands (and the other not-the-Docklands UDCs who have mostly distanced themselves smartly from LDDC policies) means substantial changes rather than merely a slightly thicker slice off the bottom of the loaf, still remains to be seen.

But the main difficulty with the accountability argument lies not so much in the demonstrable failures of UDCs to deliver – even after they have begun to profess their intention to do so – as in the inadequacies of public authority-led programmes in this sector. The two cases to which we have referred – GEAR in Glasgow and Heartlands – have both been criticised for their distant and paternalist style – for behaving, in short, as local authorities have traditionally behaved. Both tried to improve on early performance; and Heartlands now has some positive achievements to its credit – though the most impressive of these, Bloomsbury Estate Management Board, actually stems from an earlier DoE initiative (see Chapter 7). In practice, democratic accountability provides no guarantees of responsiveness, either to individuals or to local groups.

Empowerment may provide an alternative route by which regeneration can be made to yield wider benefits. However, as we saw in Chapter 10, the term itself is employed in a number of different ways. Those on the right of the political spectrum mean increasing individual autonomy and control over events. This can be secured either by an increased share of material resources, that is, wealth, or through 'top down' interventions by the central state – measures such as those proposed in John Major's 'Citizen's Charter'. As we have already seen, inner city residents have not so far gained substantially in terms of 'trickle down' from specific projects and any benefits that had accrued from general expansion in the national economy have been cut short by the disappearance of growth itself as a result of the current (1991) recession. Whether the Citizen's Charter will help to redress the balance remains to be seen; but it seems unlikely that inner city residents will be in a position to secure access to improved public services when the areas in which they live are precisely those in which persistent underfunding has compromised effective delivery of good quality public services.

It may be that new regeneration projects promoted by the private sector will provide some benefit for individuals in terms of social and environmental schemes introduced by benevolent developers. But on the evidence we have reviewed, the likelihood is that such benefit will once again be marginal: improved shopping facilities, at best; or a fistful of small grants from a community trust and some ornamental statuary to help locals feel better about being poor and powerless in newly improved surroundings.

The Left means something different by empowerment: the assumption of control by communities acting collectively. The Conservative government began the new phase of enterprise initiatives with considerable suspicions about the potential role of communities and groups acting in their name. Kenneth Clarke, when Inner Cities Minister, bracketed them with local authorities as incorrigible naysayers; he referred dismissively to 'self-appointed groups of ad-hoc spokesmen, who bog us down in a great deal of jargon politics and campaigning'. He concluded that 'In some areas, if we cannot identify any worthwhile contributions from the community we are going to have to introduce acceptable agencies' (*Employment News*, July 1986). Douglas Hurd had also added to the indictment by referring to interest group 'pressures' which 'do not necessarily add up to the general good' (speech to The Royal Institute of Public Administration 1986). The role of oppositional groups in Docklands added further weight to official disapproval. And yet, as the National Council for Voluntary Organisations had pointed out in their memorandum to ministers, voluntary action 'can pull together action, owned by local people across the divisions that separate different segments of the public and private sector' (Memo, July 1987).

Moreover, over the decade, community groups have accumulated a substantial list of examples of direct involvement in urban regeneration, culminating in the case of Coin Street (Chapter 10) where a community-led scheme has eventually been implemented. But community action by itself will only occasionally, with a special conjunction of circumstances, be sufficient and, with the rare exception of socially and ethnically homogeneous neighbourhoods, risks excluding vulnerable groups at the margin.

This leads logically to the final element: partnership. This can mean almost anything – or virtually nothing. Once it meant joint action promoted by central and local government; later, it has come to mean partnership between public and private sector, enthusiastically promoted by organisations like Business in the Community. The chief merit of the Heartlands experiment was that it furnished a working model of effective public–private sector cooperation in implementation; one of its less successful aspects has been the failure to incorporate local people fully in that process.

However, it does seem evident that as far as the broader objectives of addressing social deprivation are concerned the partnership approach is a considerable advance on either the 'pure private' or the 'single-minded' development-oriented UDC. The private sector's social input works better if the public sector sets a framework and provides the infrastructure; Bordesley Village is a vast improvement on Stockbridge. The local authority planning function earns its place as part of this process. The concept of partnership advanced by developers like Nigel Mobbs is one in which the public sector's role is to contribute resources for development with no strings attached: what people of his persuasion used to call in another context throwing public money at problems. 'British town planners are not concerned with results, only policy', he observed in his Aims of Industry pamphlet, and 'bureaucrats are perfectionists, not achievers' (Mobbs 1986: 11). This approach – developers as urban Napoleons – met its Waterloo in the shambles of Docklands' missing transport infrastructure.

But this is not to imply that the public sector partners must necessarily be the direct providers of services; here, there is scope for substantial development of the role of voluntary organisations and community groups in different forms of active partnership. So if, despite its past inadequacies, the case for local government as the pivotal organisation remains strong, especially in addressing the broader social as well as the narrower economic goals of policy, that case remains conditional. Conditional, first of all internally, upon devising a formula which facilitates the development of an active partnership with locally-based organisations of all kinds; and externally, in the evolution of working relationships with industry and with the local representatives of central government.

Whether central government now favours this kind of partnership, growing out of local circumstances rather than imposed from above, remains problematic. Plans for a massive new development corporation covering an area stretching along the banks of the Thames estuary to the east of the Docklands area have been worked up under the personal patronage of Michael Heseltine. As for local government, the Department of the Environment is currently considering schemes for structural reforms, and is meanwhile attempting to implant the enterprise culture in local authorities through the device of the City Challenge – making authorities compete for a share of inner city funding before a panel of judges consisting of DoE ministers. Public pronouncements sometimes suggest that ministers would like to be at one and the same time in a position to scapegoat local authorities for failure and claim credit for any successes. But at the minimum there seems now to be a recognition that a coherent policy requires local government's participation – on whatever terms. Whether or not the proposed urban regeneration agency (see p. 61, Note 2) will encourage such participation or serve further to exclude local government, may turn out to be as much a matter of organisational dynamics as of intended policy.

And what of the fundamental cultural changes that would ensure that the revitalisation is self-sustaining and that no more injections of public funds will be required to sustain 'hustle and bustle' in the inner cities? With the benefit of 20:20 hindsight, it can now be seen that some projects are beyond the wit even of Conservative ministers to implement. They lie buried with the failed private sector solutions of the recent past – to await resurrection in the next turn of the perpetually revolving wheel of inner city policy.

References

Aldridge, M. (1979) *The British New Towns*, London: Routledge & Kegan Paul.

Aldridge, M. and Edwards, J. (1989) *Living with Inner City Policies*, Department of Social Policy, Royal Holloway and Bedford New College.

Anson, B. (1981) *I'll Fight You For It!*, London: Jonathan Cape.

Archbishop of Canterbury's Commission on Urban Priority Areas (1985) *Faith in the City*, London: Church House Publishing.

Association of Municipal Authorities (1988) *Programme for Partnership*, London: AMA.

Aston University (1985) *Five Year Review of the Birmingham Inner City Partnership*, Birmingham: University of Aston Management Centre.

Audit Commission (1989) *Urban Regeneration and Economic Development: The Local Government Dimension*, London: HMSO.

Balchin, P. N. and Bull, G. (1987) *Regional and Urban Economics*, London: Harper & Row.

Barlow Report (1940) *Report of the Royal Commission on the Distribution of the Industrial Population*, Cmnd 6153, London: HMSO.

Barnekov, T., Boyle, R. and Rich, D. (1989) *Privatism and Urban Policy in Britain and the United States*, Oxford: Oxford University Press.

Batley, R. (1989) 'London Docklands: An Analysis of Power Relations Between UDCs and Local Government', *Public Administration*, 67(2): 167–87.

Benyon, J. and Solomos, J. (1987) *The Roots of Urban Unrest*, Oxford: Pergamon.

Birmingham City Council (1988) *Handsworth Coordinating Committee, Response to Handsworth Riots*, 13 February 1988.

Birmingham City Council (1990) *Report of Economic Development Committee*, 6 November 1990.

Birmingham City Council (1991) *Heartlands Social Strategy*, unpublished draft.

Birmingham Heartlands Ltd (1988) *A Strategy for the East Birmingham Inner City Renewal*.

Birmingham Heartlands Ltd (1989a) *Bordesley Development Framework*.

Birmingham Heartlands Ltd (1989b) *Nechells Development Framework*.

Birmingham Heartlands Ltd (1991a) *Statement of Objectives*.

Birmingham Heartlands Ltd (1991b) *Progress report*, February.

Birmingham Heartlands Community Trust (1991) *First Annual Report*.

Birmingham Inner City Partnership (1988) *Programme*, 1988/91.

Birmingham Polytechnic (1989) *Social Survey of Heartlands, 1988*, Birmingham: Birmingham Polytechnic.

Birmingham Voluntary Services Council (1989) *Child Care in East Birmingham*.

Black Country Development Corporation (1989) Annual Report.

Brindley, T., Rydin, Y. and Stoker, G. (1989) *Remaking Planning*, London: Unwin Hyman.

Brown, M. and Madge, N. (1982) *Despite the Welfare State*, London: Heinemann.

Brownill, S. (1990) *Developing London's Docklands: Another Greater Planning Disaster?*, London: Paul Chapman.

Brownrigg, M. (1983) 'Clydebank: The Economics of Decline', *The Planner*, 69(3): 85–7.

Buck, N., Gordon, G. and Young, K. (1986) *The London Employment Problem*, Oxford: Oxford University Press.

Business in the Community (1988) *The Future for Enterprise Agencies*, London: BiC.

Cabinet Office (1988) *Action for Cities*, London: Cabinet Office.

Cambridge Economic Policy Review (1982), Vol. 8, Aldershot: Gower.

Carley, M. (1981) *Social Measurement and Social Indicators*, London: George Allen & Unwin.

Centre for Local Economic Strategies (1989) *Urban Development Corporations*: Interim Monitoring report, Manchester: CLES.

Church, A. (1988) 'Urban regeneration in London's Docklands: A Five Year Policy Review', *Environment and Planning*, Vol 6: 187–206.

City of Manchester Planning Department (1982) *Manchester's Inner Area*, Manchester: City of Manchester.

Clarke, K. (1986) As quoted under 'Handsworth to be Part of £8m. Initiative on Jobs', *The Times*, 7 February.

Clarke, K. (1988) As quoted under 'Private Cash Targeted to Fund Plans for Cities', *The Independent*, 8 March.

Coffield, F., Robinson, P. and Sarsby, J. (1980) *A Cycle of Deprivation?*, London: Heinemann.

Colenutt, R. (1991) 'The London Docklands Development Corporation: Has the Community benefitted?', in Keith, M. and Rogers, A., *Hollow Promises: Rhetoric and Reality in the Inner City*, London: Mansell.

Community Development Project (1975) *Local Government Becomes Big Business*, Coventry CDP Final Report Part 2.

Community Development Project (1976) *Local Government Becomes Big Business*, CDP.

Community Development Project (1977a) *Gilding the Ghetto*, CDP.

Community Development Project (1977b) *The Costs of Industrial Change*, London: Home Office.

Confederation of British Industries (1988) *Initiatives Beyond Charity*, Report of a Task Force.

Conservative Party (1992) *The Best Future for Britain*, London: The Conservative Manifesto.

Corner, J. and Harvey, S. (1990) 'Enterprise as a Cultural Project', *Magazine of Cultural Studies*, 1, March, 24–7.

Cullingworth, J. B. (1973) *Problems of an Urban Society*, Vol 2, London: Allen & Unwin.

Cullingworth, J. B. (1985) *Town and Country Planning in Britain*, 9th Edn, London: Allen & Unwin.

Davis-Coleman, C. (1986) 'Heseltine: My faith in Urban Development Corporations', *Municipal Journal*, 24 October: 1850–1.

Dawson, J. and Parkinson, M. (1991) 'Merseyside Development Corporation, 1981–89', in Keith, M. and Rogers, A. *Hollow Promises*, London: Mansell.

Department of the Environment (1977a) *Inner London: Policies for Dispersal and Balance: Final Report of the Lambeth Inner Area Study*, London: D.O.E.

Department of the Environment (1977b) *Change and Decay: Final Report of the Liverpool Inner Area Study*, London: D.O.E.

Department of the Environment (1977c) *Unequal City: Final Report of the Birmingham Inner Area Study*, London: D.O.E.

Department of the Environment (1977d) *Liverpool, Birmingham and Lambeth Inner Area Studies: Summaries of Consultants' Final Reports*, London: D.O.E.

Department of the Environment (1977e) *Policy for the Inner Cities*, Cmnd 6845, London: HMSO.

Department of the Environment (1978) *Press Release No. 520*, 26 August, London: D.O.E.

Department of the Environment (1979) *Inner Cities Policy: Press Notice No. 390*, September, London: D.O.E.

Department of the Environment (1981a) *The Urban Programme: The Partnerships at Work*, London: D.O.E.

Department of the Environment (1981b) *Review of Inner City Policies: Press Notice No. 59*, February, London: D.O.E.

Department of the Environment (1982a) *Memorandum to the House of Commons Environment Committee H C 18–i*, London: D.O.E.

Department of the Environment (1982b) *Urban Development Grant: Guidance Notes*, London: D.O.E.

Department of the Environment (1983) *Urban Development Grant: Guidance Notes*, London: D.O.E.

Department of the Environment (1984) *Inner City Policy: England*, London: D.O.E.

Department of the Environment (1985) *Urban Programme: Management Guidance Note 2: Inner Area Programmes*, London: D.O.E.

Department of the Environment (1987) *Urban Policy and DOE Programmes*, London: D.O.E.

Department of the Environment (1988a) *Urban Policy and DOE Programmes*, London: D.O.E.

Department of the Environment (1988b) *City Grant: Guidance Notes*, London: D.O.E.

Department of the Environment (1989a) *DOE Inner City Programmes 1987–88: A Report on Achievements and Developments*, London: D.O.E.

Department of the Environment (1989b) *Progress in Cities*, London: D.O.E.

Department of the Environment (1989c) *Manchester Shopping Inquiries: Report of the Plenary Session*, London: D.O.E.

Department of the Environment (1989d) *Manchester Shopping Inquiries: Report of the Sector Session*, London: D.O.E.

Department of the Environment (1989e) *Proposed Shopping Developments in Salford and Trafford: Decision Letter*, London: D.O.E.

Department of the Environment (1990a) *Renewing the Cities*, London: D.O.E.

Department of the Environment (1990b) *People in Cities*, London: D.O.E.

Department of the Environment and Department of Employment (1987) *Action for Cities: Building on Initiative*, London D.O.E./D.O.Emp.

Department of the Environment, Department of Trade and Industry and Department of Employment (1987) *City Action Team: Your City and Your Government*, London: D.O.E./D.T.I./D.O.Emp.

Department of Trade and Industry (1989) *Task Forces in Action.*

Dicken, P. and Lloyd, P.E. (1978) 'Inner Metropolitan Industrial Change, Enterprise Structures and Policy Issues: Case Studies of Manchester and Merseyside', *Regional Studies*, 12: 181–98.

Docklands Consultative Committee (1987) *Six Year Review of the LDDC*, London: LDCC.

Docklands Consultative Committee (1990) *The Docklands Experiment: A Critical Review of Eight Years of the LDDC*, London: LDCC.

Docklands Consultative Committee (1991) *How the Cake was Cut: The Years of Docklands*, London: LDCC.

Docklands Joint Committee (1976) *London Docklands: A Strategic Plan.*

Donnison, D. V. and Middleton, A. (eds) (1987) *Regenerating the Inner City: Glasgow's Experience*, Routledge & Kegan Paul.

Edwards, J. (1981) 'Subjectivist Approaches to the Study of Social Policy Making', *Journal of Social Policy*, 10(3): 289–310.

Edwards, J. (1984) 'U.K. Inner Cities: Problem Construction and Policy Response', *Cities*, 1(6): 592–604.

Edwards, J. (1987a) *Greater Manchester Retail Inquiry: Plenary Session: Proof of Evidence*, Manchester: Ship Canal Company.

Edwards, J. (1987b) *Greater Manchester Retail Inquiry: Sector Session: Proof of Evidence*, Manchester: Ship Canal Company.

Edwards, J. and Batley, R. (1978) *The Politics of Positive Discrimination*, London: Tavistock.

Elias, P. and Keogh, G. (1982) 'Industrial Decline and Unemployment in the Inner City Areas of Great Britain: A Review of the Evidence', *Urban Studies*, 19: 1–15.

Essen, J. and Wedge, P. (1982) *Continuities in Childhood Disadvantage*, London: Heinemann.

Eversley, D. (1980) 'Employment for the Inner City', *Institute of British Geographers: Transactions: New Series*, 5(2): 141–50.

Faith, N. (1991) 'Perilous Path to a Grand Design', *Independent on Sunday*, 11 August: 12–13.

Fothergill, S. and Gudgin, G. (1982) *Unequal Growth: Urban and Regional Employment Change in the UK*, London: Heinemann.

Glancey, J. (1991) 'Gotham City, E14', *Independent*, 13 July.

Goddard, J. B. and Champion, A. G. (eds) (1983) *The Urban and Regional Transformation of Britain*, London: Methuen.

Greater Manchester Council (1986) *Greater Manchester Structure Plan.*

Greater Manchester Council Planning Department (1983) *Economic and Social Problem Areas: Policy Background Paper 83/7.*

Greater Manchester Council Planning Department (1985) *Multiple Deprivation in Greater Manchester, Policy Background Paper 85/13.*

Greve, J. (1973) *Community Development in the Context of Urban Deprivation* (paper prepared for the European Study Group in Community Development and Urban Deprivation), Oxford: United Nations Division of Social Affairs.

Gripaios, P. (1977) 'Industrial Decline in London: an Examination of its Causes', *Urban Studies*, 14.

Hadfield, P. (1988) 'Confidence is Key to Success' (interview), *Trafford Park News Magazine*, 2, Trafford Park Development Corporation.

Hadfield, P. (1990) 'January Profile', quoted in *Trafford Park Today*, Issue 1, January, Trafford Park Development Corporation.

Hall, P. (ed.) (1981) *The Inner City in Context*, London: Heinemann.

Hall, P., Thomas, R., Gracey, H. and Drewett, R. (1973) *The Containment of Urban England*, London: Allen & Unwin.

Halsey, A. H. (ed.) (1972) *Educational Priority*, London: HMSO.

Hansard, House of Commons, Vol 87 (1983) *New Urban Initiatives*, Col. 159, London: HMSO.

Hansard, House of Commons, Vol 52 (1984) *Urban Development Corporations*, Col. 118, London: HMSO.

Hansard, House of Commons, Vol 96 (1986), Col. 100, London: HMSO.

Harvey, D. (1973) *Social Justice and the City*, London: Edward Arnold.

Hatch, S., Fox, E. and Legg, C. (1977) *Research and Reform*, London: Home Office.

Hausner, V. A. (1987) *Urban Economic Change*, Oxford: Clarendon Press.

Healey, M. J. and Clark, D. (1983) 'Industrial Change in Coventry 1974-82', *City of Coventry Economic Monitor*, 4(83): 51–66.

Heclo, H. and Wildavsky, A. (1974) *The Private Government of Public Money*, London: Macmillan.

Heiser, Sir T. (1990) In House of Commons: *Committee of Public Accounts: Regenerating the Inner Cities: Thirty Third Report*, London: HMSO.

Hennessy, P. (1989) *Whitehall*, London: Fontana.

Henschel, P. (1989) *Report of talk on Public and Private Partnership in Urban Regeneration*, Royal Institute of Public Administration Report, 10 (4): 516.

Heseltine, M. (1987) *Where There's a Will*, London: Hutchinson.

Higgins, J. (1978) *The Poverty Business: Britain and America*, Oxford: Blackwell.

Higgins, J., Deakin, N., Edwards, J. and Wicks, M. (1983) *Government and Urban Poverty*, Oxford: Blackwell.

Hills, J. and Sutherland, H. (1991) 'The Proposed Council Tax', *Fiscal Studies*, 12(4): 1–21.

Holman, R. (ed) (1970) *Socially Deprived Families in Britain*, London: Bedford Square Press.

Holman, R. (1978) *Poverty: Explanations of Social Deprivation*, London: Martin Robertson.

Holtermann, S. (1975) 'Areas of Urban Deprivation in Great Britain: An Analysis of the 1971 Census Data', *Social Trends*, 6: 33–47.

Holtermann, S. (1978) 'The Welfare Economics of Priority Area Policies', *Journal of Social Policy*, 7(1): 141–56.

Home, R. (1982) *Inner City Regeneration*, London: Spon.

Home Office (1974) *Urban Programme Circular No.11*, London: Home Office.

House of Commons (1983) *White Paper: Regional Industrial Development*, Cmnd 9111, London: HMSO.

House of Commons (1990) *Committee of Public Accounts: Regenerating the Inner Cities: Thirty Third Report*, London: HMSO.

House of Commons Employment Committee (1988a) HC327-1, *The Employment Effects of Urban Development Corporations*, Employment Committee Third Report, London: HMSO.

House of Commons Employment Committee (1988b) HC327-11, *The Employment Effects of Urban Development Corporations*, Employment Committee Third Report, Minutes of Evidence, London: HMSO.

House of Commons Environment Committee (1982–3) *Memorandum by the Department of the Environment*: 501–10, London: HMSO.

Howe, Sir G. (1978) *Liberating Free Enterprise: A New Experiment*, Speech to Bow Group, June (Extracts reprinted as 'Throw the Inner Cities Wide Open to Initiative'), *Estates Times*, 512: 10–11.

Johnston, R. J. (1980) *City and Society*, Harmondsworth: Penguin.

Keith, M. and Rogers, A. (1991) *Rhetoric and Reality in the Inner City*, London: Mansell.

Kettle, M. and Hodges, L. (1982) *Uprising! The Police, the People and Riots in Britain's Cities*, London: Pan Books.

Kirby, P. (1988) 'Travelling Light in Trafford Park', *Trafford Park News Magazine*, 3: 12, Trafford Park Development Corporation.

Knox, P. (1982) *Urban Social Geography*, London: Longman.

Lansley, S. (1979) 'Rate Support Grant and the Inner Cities', *Centre for Environmental Studies Review*, 6: 56–63.

Lawless, P. (1979) *Urban Deprivation and Government Initiative*, London: Faber & Faber.

Lawless, P. (1981) *Britain's Inner Cities*, London: Harper & Row.

Lawless, P. (1988a) 'Urban Development Corporations and Their Alternatives', *Cities*, 5(3): 277–89.

Lawless, P. (1988b) 'British Urban Policy Post 1979: A critique'. *Policy and Politics*, 16(4): 261–75.

Lawless, P. and Brown, F. (1986) *Urban Growth and Change in Britain*, London: Harper & Row.

Lever, W. and Moore, C. (1986) *The City in Transition*, Oxford: Oxford University Press.

London Docklands Development Corporation (1989a) *LDDC Census of Employment*, London: LDDC.

London Docklands Development Corporation (1989b) *Social Housing Strategy*, London: LDDC.

London Docklands Development Corporation (1990a) *Annual Report and Accounts 1989/90*, London: LDDC.

London Docklands Development Corporation (1990b) *Corporate Plan*, London: LDDC.

London Docklands Development Corporation (1991) *Newsletter*, April, London: LDDC.

Loney, M. (1981) 'The British Community Development Projects: Questioning the State', *Community Development Journal*, 16(1).

Loney, M. (1983) *Community Against Government*, London: Heinemann.

MacGregor, S. (1981) *The Politics of Poverty*, London: Longman.

Mackintosh, A. and Wainwright, H. (1987) *A Taste of Power*, London: Verso.

Manchester/Salford Partnership (1985/6) *Annual Report 1985/86.*

Manchester/Salford Partnership (1989) *Manchester Inner Area Programme 1987/88–1988/89.*

Manchester Ship Canal Company (1987) *Outline Planning Application – The Trafford Centre*, Trafford: M.S.C.C.

Manners, G. (1986) 'Decentralising London, 1945–1975', in Clout, H. and Wood, P. (eds), *London: Problems of Change*, Harlow: Longman.

Marris, P. (1982) *Community Planning and Conceptions of Change*, London: Routledge & Kegan Paul.

Marsland, D. (1991) 'Squalor', *Social Policy and Administration*, 25(1): 49–62.

Merry, C. (1987) *Greater Manchester Retail Inquiry: Sector Session: Proof of Evidence*, Trafford Borough Council.

Merseyside Development Corporation (1990), *Annual Report 1989/90*.

Metcalfe, L. and Richards, S. (1987), *Improving Public Management*, London: Sage.

Mobbs, N. (1986) *The Inner Urban Challenge*, London: Aims of Industry.

Nabarro, R. and Richards, D. (1980) *Wasteland*, London: Thames Television.

National Audit Office (1988) *Report by the Comptroller and Auditor General: Development of the Environment: Urban Development Corporations*, London: HMSO.

National Audit Office (1990) *Report by the Comptroller and Auditor General: Regenerating the Inner Cities*, London: HMSO.

Nicholson, G. (1989) 'A Model of How Not to Regenerate an Urban Area', *Town and Country Planning*, 58(2): 52–5.

PA/Cambridge Economic Consultants (1989) *The Government's Handsworth Task Force: An Evaluation Report*, London: DTI.

PA/Cambridge Economic Consultants (1991a) *An Evaluation of the Government's Inner Cities Task Force Initiative*, Summary Report, London: DTI.

PA/Cambridge Economic Consultants (1991b) *An Evaluation of the Government's Inner Cities Task Force Initiative, Volume Four: Handsworth Task Force*, London: DTI.

Parkinson, M. and Duffy, J. (1984) 'The Minister for Merseyside and the Task Force', *Parliamentary Affairs*, 37(1): 76–96.

Peat Marwick McLintock (1986) *The Impact of Canary Wharf*, unpublished Report for LDDC.

PE/Inbucon (1989) *East Birmingham Skills Survey*, Birmingham: East Birmingham Task Force.

Policy Studies Institute (1991) *Company Investment in the Community*, London: PSI.

Pryce, K, (1979) *Endless Pressure*, Harmondsworth: Penguin.

Rees, G. and Lambert, R. (1985) *Cities in Crisis*, London: Edward Arnold.

Rex, J. (1988) *The Ghetto and the Underclass*, Aldershot: Avebury.

Ridge, M. and Smith, B. (1990) 'The First Months of the Community Charge', *Fiscal Studies*, 11(3): 39–54.

Robinson, W. S. (1950) 'Ecological Correlations and the Behaviour of Individuals', *American Sociological Review*, XV: 351–7.

Robson, B. (1987) *Greater Manchester Retail Inquiry: Plenary Session: Proof of Evidence*, Greater Manchester Consortium.

Robson, B. (1988) *Those Inner Cities*, Oxford: Clarendon Press.

Rutter, M. and Madge, N. (1976) *Cycles of Disadvantage*, London: Heinemann.

Salford City Council (1987a) *Rule 6 Statement of Proposed Submission by Salford City Council to the Public Inquiry: The Regatta Centre*.

Salford City Council (1987b) *A Plan for Jobs*.

Schaffer, F. (1972) *The New Town Story*, London: Paladin.

Shields, M. (1988) 'Urban Regeneration and Development Corporations: A Reply to Parkinson', *Local Economy*, 3(3): 201–4.

Shields, M. (1990) 'Chief Executive's Review', *Trafford Park Development Corporation Annual Report 1989–1990*, Trafford Park Development Corporation.

Shields, M. (1991) 'Comment', *Profile and Property News*, Spring, Trafford Park Development Corporation.

Sills, A., Taylor, G. and Golding, P. (1988) *The Politics of the Urban Crisis*, London: Hutchinson.

Skeffington Report (1969) *Report of the Committee on Public Participation in Planning: People and Planning*, London: HMSO.

Smith, S. and Squire, D. (1986) 'The Local Government Green Paper', *Fiscal Studies*, 7(2): 63–71.

Solesbury, W. (1987) 'Urban Policy in the 1980s: The Issues and Arguments', *The Planner*, 73 (6): 18–22.

Southern, C. (1990) 'January Profile: Peter Hadfield', *Trafford Park Today*, Issue 1, January, Trafford Park Development Corporation.

Specht, H. (1976) *The Community Development Project*, London: National Institute for Social Work Papers No.2.

Spence, N. A. and Frost, M. E. (1983) 'Urban Employment Change', in Goddard, J. B. and Champion, A. G. (eds), *The Urban and Regional Transformation of Britain*, London: Methuen.

Spencer, K., Taylor, A., Smith, B., Mawson, J., Flynn, N. and Batley, R. (1986) *Crisis in the Industrial Heartland: A Study of the West Midlands*, Oxford: Clarendon Press.

Stocks, N. (1987a) *Greater Manchester Retail Inquiry: Plenary Session: Proof of Evidence*, Trafford Borough Council.

Stocks, N. (1987b) *Greater Manchester Retail Inquiry: Sector Session: Proof of Evidence*, Trafford Borough Council.

Stoker, G. (1989) 'Urban Development Corporations: A Review', *Regional Studies* 23(2): 159–73.

Struthers, W. (1987) *Greater Manchester Retail Inquiry: Sector Session: Proof of Evidence*, Salford City Council.

Tibbott, R. (1987) *Greater Manchester Retail Inquiry: Sector Session: Proof of Evidence*, London: Leisure and Recreation Consultants.

Titmuss, R. (1968) *Commitment to Welfare*, London: Allen & Unwin.

Townsend, P. (1976) 'The Difficulties of Policies Based on the Concept of Area Deprivation', Barnett Shine Foundation Lecture, Queen Mary College, University of London.

Townsend, P. (1987) *Greater Manchester Retail Inquiry: Plenary Session: Proof of Evidence*, Greater Manchester Consortium.

Trafford (1987a) *Rule 6 Statement of Proposed Submission by the Trafford Borough Council to the Public Inquiry: The Trafford Centre*, Trafford Borough Council.

Trafford (1987b) *Rule 6 Statement of Proposed Submission by the Trafford Borough Council to the Public Inquiry: Westside Park*, Trafford Borough Council.

Trafford Park Development Corporation (1987) *The Trafford Centre: Planning Appeal at Dumplington Trafford (Letter to Secretary of State for the Environment)*, Trafford Park Development Corporation.

Trafford Park Development Corporation (1988a) *Corporate Plan*.

Trafford Park Development Corporation (1988b) 'Kellogg's Sets Standard for Park Partnership', *Trafford Park News Magazine*, 3: 4.

Trafford Park Development Corporation (1988c) 'Highways', *Trafford Park News Magazine*, 2.

Trafford Park Development Corporation (1988d) *Consultation Code*.

Trafford Park Development Corporation (1989a) *Trafford Park: Where Businesses Work.*
Trafford Park Development Corporation (1989b) 'Kellogg's – Committed to Trafford Park', *Regional Development*, September.
Trafford Park Development Corporation (1989c) *City Link: Public Briefing.*
Trafford Park Development Corporation (1989d) *Parkway/M602 Link: Public Briefing.*
Trafford Park Development Corporation (1989e) *Labour Market Survey.*
Trafford Park Development Corporation (1990a) *Trafford Park: Greater Manchester.*
Trafford Park Development Corporation (1990b) *Annual Report 1st April 1989–31st March 1990.*
Trafford Park Development Corporation (1990c) *Where Businesses Work.*
Trafford Park Development Corporation (1990d) *Annual Report 1989–1990.*
Trafford Park Development Corporation (1990e) 'Trafford Park Village Plan is the People's Choice', *Trafford Park News Magazine*, 4.
Trafford Park Development Corporation (1991a) *Current Social Community Initiatives.*
Trafford Park Development Corporation (1991b) *Progress Report.*
Trafford Park Development Corporation (1991c) *Proposed Shopping Developments in Salford and Trafford: Representation to the Secretary of State for the Environment.*
Trafford Park Industrial Council (1990) 'From the Secretary's Desk', *Traffic News*, Spring.
Trafford Park Investment Strategy (1986) *Trafford Park Investment Strategy: Final Report*, London: Roger Tym and Partners.
Travers Morgan Partnership (1973) *Docklands Study Report*, London.
Trippier, D. (1988) 'Quay West Brings a Hint of Dallas to Wharfside', quoted in *Trafford Park News Magazine*, 4.
Turok, I. (1987) 'Lessons for Local Economic Policy', in Donnison, D. and Middleton, A. (eds), *Regenerating the Inner City*, London: Routledge & Kegan Paul.
Tym, R. (1987a) *Birmingham Heartlands: Development Strategy for East Birmingham*, mimeo, London: Roger Tym and Partners.
Tym, R. (1987b) *Greater Manchester Retail Inquiry: Plenary Session: Proof of Evidence*, London: Roger Tym and Partners.
Vulliamy, E. (1988) 'A Wider Wealth', *Guardian*, 6 January.
Ward, C. (1989) *Welcome. Thinner City*, London: Bedford Square Press.
Wedge, P. and Prosser, N. (1973) *Born to Fail?* London: Arrow Books.
West Midlands County Council (1986) *A Different Reality: Report of the Review Panel on the Handsworth Rebellion* (Silverman Report), Birmingham: Birmingham and West Midlands County Council.
Whitting, G. (1985) *Implementing an Inner City Policy*, School for Advanced Urban Studies Occasional Paper, 22, Bristol: SAUS.
Whyatt, A. (1988) 'The Prospects for Local Economic and Employment Policy: Towards a More Coherent Approach', *Local Economy*, 3(2): 126–31.
Widgery, D. (1991) *Some Lives!: A GP's East End*, London: Sinclair-Stevenson.
Williams, W. (1988) *Washington, Westminster and Whitehall*, Cambridge: Cambridge University Press.
Wolfenden Report (1978) *The Future of Voluntary Organisations*, London: Croom Helm.
Wolmar, C. (1989) 'The New East Enders', *Guardian*, 8–9 April: 1–5.

Name index

Subject index